MW01290298

SEX POSITIONS

Tips and Techniques to Master Amazing Sex Positions

Crystal Hardie & Rick Reynolds

© Copyright 2016 - All rights reserved.

In no way is it legal to reproduce, duplicate, or transmit any part of this document in either electronic means or in printed format. Recording of this publication is strictly prohibited and any storage of this document is not allowed unless with written permission from the publisher. All rights reserved.

The information provided herein is stated to be truthful and consistent, in that any liability, in terms of inattention or otherwise, by any usage or abuse of any policies, processes, or directions contained within is the solitary and utter responsibility of the recipient reader. Under no circumstances will any legal responsibility or blame be held against the publisher for any reparation, damages, or monetary loss due to the information herein, either directly or indirectly.
Respective authors own all copyrights not held by the publisher.

Legal Notice:
This book is copyright protected. This is only for personal use. You cannot amend, distribute, sell, use, quote or paraphrase any part or the content within this book without the consent of the author or copyright owner. Legal action will be pursued if this is breached.

Disclaimer Notice:
Please note the information contained within this document is for educational and entertainment purposes only. Every attempt has been made to provide accurate, up to date and reliable complete information. No warranties of any kind are expressed or implied. Readers acknowledge that the author is not engaging in the rendering of legal, financial, medical or professional advice.

By reading this document, the reader agrees that under no circumstances are we responsible for any losses, direct or indirect, which are incurred as a result of the use of information contained within this document, including, but not limited to, —errors, omissions, or inaccuracies.

Table of Contents

Introduction

When Dr. Alex Comfort published his 1972 book, *The Joy of Sex*, all hell broke loose. The world was not quite ready for the proposition that sex was supposed to be fun. In fact, for American religious zealots of the day, sex was no fun at all and a matter to be discussed only in the privacy of a darkened bedroom. And so it was that the nascent Religious Right movement demanded that the book be removed from libraries all across the nation.

This, however, did not prevent *The Joy of Sex* from dominating the bestseller list for quite some time. Someone certainly read it, despite the best efforts of zealots to suppress it. Never mind the fact that it remained in the top five for a full seventy weeks in the two years following publication. In other words, it was a national sensation.

When we think of that period of time, perhaps we remember Richard Nixon, Watergate, the oil crisis and maybe even the Vietnam War. Perhaps we remember *all* those historic cataclysms, but through the lens of the waning years of the Hippie Revolution.

The Christian "conservative" movement in the United States began to take root and grow, at least in part, because of the youth, civil rights and women's rights movements in the 1960s. Hot on the heels of the Beat Generation, came the white-picket-fence's antithesis – lives lived without boundaries and without rules previously believed to be the gold standard for all. It was all so improper. So wild and unhinged. So hairy. So sexy. So un-American.

The counter-Revolution would continue apace and to this day, remains a political force. While greatly diminished, what was later to take on the moniker "Moral Majority" raised to what it saw as the challenge of sexual openness, experimentation with drugs and the sheer horror of women escaping from their appointed positions in the kitchen. The era of Don Draper and his *Mad Men* was over and it seemed America was growing up too quickly for the taste of some, as the wheel turned and history marched on.

All this is the backdrop for *The Joy of Sex* and the great, American duality of purpose – to be both a beacon unto the nations and the Spanish Inquisition, simultaneously. It's true there's a segment of society that continues to insist that the darkened bedrooms of the nation are the only place for a discussion about sex and sexuality. It's also true that it's this same segment which insists on poking its head through that bedroom door to see what we're up to in there and who we're doing it with.

Duality of purpose is a funny thing.

Despite the efforts of those who fear that somewhere, someone may be having a good time (hat tip, H.L. Mencken), time has most mercifully marched on. Today, we find ourselves living in a world of sexual openness and possibility and the acceptance of those who differ from us in their sexual orientations and gender perceptions. These are good changes. These are needed changes.

But banality has set in. Sexuality has become a perfunctory and mundane affair. Even the Hippies, with their long hair and tie-dyed Bacchanalian sexual attitudes, probably knew it would all come crashing down on them, in the end. Many of them figured it out only when they looked out their kitchen windows and realized – "This is no acid flashback, man. I really *am* in Colorado Springs." Perhaps we can trace the demise of sex in our times to the satyr-like womanizing of Abbie Hoffman, or the marriage of the former *Barbarella* (of Orgasmatron fame) Jane Fonda and Tom Hayden. Whenever it happened, though, sex became the frozen condensed orange juice of our personal lives. Something we mixed up and hoped would not foul our sense of flavor.

Whatever it was that triggered the demise of satisfying, lasting sexual connections, it's lead to this latter day banality. It's refried (and not in that good, *frijoles* way). It's reconstituted, ersatz, bland, boring slurry, stuffed in our faces at every turn. There it is, staring us down, daring us to tell it how many times per week we "do it". Less than three times? Unhealthy!

Breasts loom from push up bras, twenty feet high, towering over us menacingly. Shirtless males leer at us in the latest must have jeans. Salacious tales of politicians tapping their feet in bathroom stalls and wearing diapers with women they rent, scream at us from the headlines of newspapers. But the internet has it all beat.

On the internet, one can order in sex! Just like Chinese food and only slightly less cost effective. Men can observe partially dressed (or nude) women performing various sex acts with objects, other women, men or a combination of all of the above. Pornography can be had in black and white, color, still photography, film, video, or live streamed feed. It's all there and it's all monotonously banal. We are duly saturated with it.

It seems that people have come to prefer sex that doesn't involve the presence of another human being. Even order-in sex can't hope to compete with the US pornography industry, which rakes in an almost inconceivable $10 billion to $12 billion per year, in the USA, alone. Interestingly, the constituency that appears to consume it most voraciously is the same one that rose in reaction to the morally permissive Hippies. In a 2014 survey, 50% of men who had recently attended a Promise Keepers (men's revival) rally, admitted to having viewed pornography, within one week of having done so. From Jesus to group sex in 60 seconds and all in the privacy of their own homes.

Nonetheless, the effect on our sex lives is to leave us even less satisfied than we were in the days before Dr. Comfort broke the barrier between the darkened bedroom and the town square, where sexual openness is concerned. Repression has been replaced with saturation. Prudery replaced with banality. Sex has gone from being fun to being boring and that, to me at least, is a sad state of affairs.

So I'm writing this book as a love letter to those of you who are feeling the deep freeze between the sexes in the midst of this glut of sexual openness, wondering why you don't enjoy it more, now that you're no longer chained by the bonds of moral propriety. In a time in which we should all be enjoying our sexuality with unmitigated glee, we struggle. Heterosexual people, particularly, are having more difficulty connecting. They're also having much more difficulty finding enduring relationships. Some of this is due to the commodification of sex.

Why buy the cow if you can get the milk for free? Why buy the pig for the sake of a little sausage? In a worldwide marketplace, it can seem futile. But if we're really invested in our relationships, then we're willing to do what it takes to make them work and the hinge of our loving relationships is, of course, sex.

Sex binds us together, physically. While not necessarily the most important reality in our relationships, we all have to admit to ourselves that our initial impulses toward our partners were sexual. Where do those impulses go, when the fire goes out? Can they ever be recovered? Or are they lost forever, in the whirl of cam girls, smooth-chested boys in tight jeans and looming, twenty-foot-high breasts, perfectly lifted and squashed together to render them as menacingly fleshly as possible?

My answer to that is a firm "no". But a lot of that depends on you. You bought this book, so I'm willing to bet you'll agree with that answer and that you're willing to do what it takes to re-kindle the fire and get it roaring once again. This book is dedicated to the recovery of our sex lives – all of us, wherever we are. The reclamation of genuine, flesh and blood human sexuality is something I believe in and something, further, that I believe can change the world and make it a better place.

Let's find out how you and your partner can re-kindle the flame of lust between you, by going out on a sexual limb to get at the sweetest fruit. It's never too late. The raw material is still there and that raw material is love.

Chapter 1: Where Did All the Good Times Go?

Marriage, at the best of times, is a challenge. With women now (ostensibly) on an equal footing with men, men feel a little challenged. The dynamic, for the most part, has shifted. That dynamic is one based on power and when power is diffused across previously existing boundaries, it's far less potent. It's in the hands of more of us now, and so men grope their way forward, feeling as though they've been knocked down the sexual totem pole. Where once lived a lion, now lives a lamb – at least in terms of the perception of some of my brethren.

It's natural to feel wistful for the days of *Mad Men*, if you grew up with a meatloaf-wielding mom, neat apron ever in place. But for the young men of today, living in a 24/7 sexual marketplace, negotiating relationships with living women is a matter of swiping left, or right. Tinder and other hook up apps and online dating marketplaces have made relationships between young men and women more impersonal and perfunctory (and banal) than they've ever been.

Just add to all this to the nature of marriage itself. The arrangement is intended to be monogamous and life long. Life long monogamy. It's a wonder people take on the commission any more. Maybe it's because a lot of people get married in the fiery furnace of passion that accompanies the first rosy blush of love. This is the tradition. We are intended, due to religious prescription, to abstain from sex prior to marriage. While few of us do any longer, it's clear that many of us enter into marriage in a sex haze that is no reflection (at all) of reality. Many of us tend to overlook the "forever" part, or just believe that the passion will endure. For some it does – effortlessly. For most? Not so much.

Many of us these days choose co-habitation as our version of monogamy. Sometimes, it works. Sometimes, serial monogamy becomes a lifelong habit to the point that we contemplate, at some point, the installation of a revolving door. But whether we choose to obtain an institutional stamp of approval for our union, or to bypass that part and make a horizontal move to co-habitation, we all like to believe it's going to last.

So this book is geared to those of us in marital relationships and especially – to those of us in heterosexual relationships. It's not that I want to exclude anybody. It's just that what I see around me is sending the message that the het population is having a very tough time with sexual identity. Things don't seem quite as cut and dried as they once were, for one. Evolving gender presumptions have eroded, along with their accompanying roles. The commodified sex market is ever present, threatening the whole idea of life long, romantic lover. Online dating and hook up apps are just a little too convenient not to tempt many.

If the recent Ashley Madison scandal taught us anything, it's that a lot of people are looking for extra-marital sexual activity. I guess we all knew that, but the nature of the scandal pointed out exactly how widespread this tendency is. It can be found in the halls of power and the Sports Hall of Fame. In the military, it can be found from Generals right down to the Private on latrine duty. From the prim school teacher to the high-powered CEO, bored with her husband – people are getting busy with people they aren't married to.

In the USA, where half of all marriages are doomed to failure, 41% of married couples admit to infidelity. Of this number, 57% of men admit to extra-curricular activity, while 54% of women do. So it seems the naughty is rather evenly distributed between the sexes. New statistics relate also relate that people under thirty are more likely to cheat on their partners than ever before.

That "room mate" thing

It creeps up on you. It slinks around the house, perhaps manifesting itself in a pair of socks stuffed between the couch cushions, or an unwashed bra lying on the floor, abandoned. Sweat pants with holes in them. Unshaven faces and armpits. Suddenly Netflix and chill is more about who polishes off the lion's share of the popcorn, than who makes the first move.

Where once you longed to see each other, rushing home to those loving arms, now you amble in the front door and greet each other wanly, thinking "Oh. You again?" We hate to admit it. It's sad and pathetic. Sooner or later, though, most married or long term monogamous couples become roommates. Still loving each other, we're no longer surprised by a stray fart (regardless of how loud, or odorous) and leave the bathroom door open when taking a dump (and we call it exactly that, to each other's faces).

It's almost inevitable.

Sex is a brokered situation. One of you turns to the other and says, "Wanna' have sex?" The question hangs in the air, limply appealing. Finally, the other answers, "Tonight?"

Roommates.

Saturday night was once your inviolable sex appointment. With a nice, long sleep in between you and a busy week, this would be your "do or die" nooky night. No outs. No excuses. But then, the Saturdays would start to come and go and no one would seem to remember when Saturday night stopped meaning something. Pretty soon, a month will have gone by...then six weeks. Etcetera.

Is this really any way to live, as two people who not so long ago couldn't keep their hands off each other? Are you going to spend the rest of your sexless lives gazing off into space, thinking "what if", or going the Ashley Madison, or Tinder route and lying to each other about it?

Those are the standard solutions called upon to remediate heterosexual bed death, but they're easy ways out that lead to structural demise. They usually lead to the revolving door, whether you're married or not.

The solution is right in front of your face and it's your

partner. Why are you living together if you never have sex with each other? To share the rent? While the society we live in encourages passive observation, quick fixes and short attention spans, some things are worth saving. If you're willing to do what's required and you think it's worth the effort, then I suggest you keep reading.

Men, you're going to need to shave for this. Women, you too. Ladies and gentlemen – start your razors.

Chapter 2: Do You Remember the Time?

The first kiss is like a slow blooming flower of revelation. You may have been stalking one another for a while, looking for excuses to "bump into" each other. Or you may have seen each other across a crowded room and fallen straight into the velvet abyss of the sex haze that descended immediately thereafter.

That moment is the moment you decided there was a connection, because that first kiss is what really decides who stays and who goes. Everything else is built on it. That's because when people kiss each other on the mouth; when their lips linger, they're displaying their sexual interest in one another. Kissing on the mouth is easily as intimate as sexual intercourse and is, in fact, its precursor. The quality of that first kiss is very often a solid indication of the quality of sex to come.

Part of getting back to the sexuality you once shared as a "starter" couple is remembering what it was that set you off in the first place. What was it about your partner that first attracted you? Was it physical appearance? A sense of humor? A hat tilted at a jaunty angle? Maybe it was a unique laugh that now grates on your nerves a bit (so forget that one).

Focus on whatever that was and ask yourself, is that the quality what made you stay? It doesn't matter what the answer to the question is. The answer is less important than drilling down into your shared past and remembering a feeling as accurately as you can.

My story

When I first met the love of my life, I was alone, in a foreign country. Situations like that can make one vulnerable to some pretty serious mistakes. But there was something about her as she came though the door of the nightclub I was visiting in Prague. She literally danced through the door, winning my heart with a few flawless moves, before I had any clear idea what she actually looked like. "You're on vacation", I thought to myself. "You'll probably never see her again, so don't get yourself going, buddy."

I lost track of her for a while, after that first glimpse of the woman who'd come to be the meaning of the word "love" to me. Later that evening, though, she approached my table and asked if she might sit down. She didn't know she'd had me at "dancing through the door". She hadn't noticed me there, in the darkness. But as though by some universal force, there she was, this vivacious creature, smiling at me from across the table. Again, I thought, "You're on vacation, buddy."

She was English. I was American. It was impossible and we

knew it. Then, we didn't know it. We had no idea what we'd become. We visited each other, taking turns to fly back and forth and finally, we realized we were doing it "wrong". We knew that the real self-deception wasn't stringing out a one-night stand into a relationship. It was ignoring the earth-shattering significance of what had really happened – two worlds colliding in an explosion of recognition. She was "the one". I was "the one". This was "it".

And she is exactly who that little dance told me she was, that first night of knowing we were each on the earth, so long ago. It's very clear to both of us (now, anyways) that the cosmos conspired to draw us into each other's arms. But that doesn't mean the ride isn't bumpy sometimes. It doesn't mean we don't fight, or have taken each other a little for granted as time has passed. That can happen to even the most star-crossed of lovers; that roommate thing and we are no exception.

But the memory of that night and the fact we found each other in a distant land and somehow ended up in each other's presence has never dimmed. We both cleave to that moment as our creation myth – the establishment of the essence of "us" and that is our glue. But that glue continues to be reinforced by our sex life.

That doesn't mean to say we spend every waking moment cooking up new ways to turn each other on, or to bring novelty into our bedroom. We know that sex, while an important part of any loving couple's life, is not intended to dominate one's life. Who would ever get anything done? We know it waxes and wanes in intensity and that, sometimes, partners aren't as in sync in terms of libido, as they might like to be. That's true of pretty well everyone else I can think of. What we also understand, though, is that we need to feed each other. We need to keep in mind, at all times, that our carnality (the fleshy, sensual part of us) is an opportunity to strengthen and fortify our bond through the physical act of love.

Sex is a demonstration. Saying "I love you" is a demonstration of another kind. Together, these demonstrations form a powerful complex of supportive and enduring love that means business and stands the test of time. So we "remember the time when we fell in love" (as Michael Jackson once sang), as often as possible. The commemoration of that blissful, mythical night is, in fact, the anniversary we celebrate together, each and every year. We've even been back to Prague on one or two of the milestones of our time together to do it in high, romantic style.

There's that word. Romance. Sex and romance, in a loving relationship are absolutely indivisible. These two are the twin concepts that form "the beast with two backs" in the context of a long-term partnership or marriage. You can't have one without the other. That's why the sweatpants and all its inconsiderate little buddies need to be kept to a dull roar in your marriage/partnership. To be with one another and to be totally present to your romantic history (as a present reality in your relationship), you can't let that roommate thing win.

Sex positions are myriad, but their basis is a combination of factors. We've talked about defining qualities as a touchstone for re-establishing sexual connection. Now we should talk about daily life and the many opportunities for expressing our love, which pass us by, unnoticed, every day.

They're waiting for you to exploit them and to reap the benefits they can bring to your ongoing love affair with your partner.

Chapter 3: Clearing the Decks for Sex

Sex isn't something you should just "count on". That's one thing my love and I have learned over the years. For us, the initial fire hasn't so much gone out as it had to be domesticated and kept in its proper place. To be truthful, that's because we entered into our relationship with a strong awareness of how tenuous love can be. We were both committed to maintaining the quality of our bond and that meant a frank and open discussion about our sex life together, once the initial madness of love had subsided.

You know what it's like. You can't keep your hands off each other. You can barely be in the same room together, without "going there". People yell "Get a room!" at you in the street, because you're always smooching (and proudly so). Exhibitionism and day and night eroticism fuel the early bonding of all couples. Keeping that feeling alive, though, when life interrupts your mutual sexual reverie, can be a demanding and serious undertaking.

Tempus fugit (time flies)

It's no secret that the fast-paced nature of life can get in the way of our sex lives. This is especially true if you have children (babies and very young children, especially). The demands of child rearing present their own challenges. But that's not really the focus of this book. Let's focus on ways and means of making sure you're not putting your sexuality on the backburner out of sheer laziness, cavalier neglect, or just exhaustion.

Sex in a long-term partnership can dwindle in many ways and being aware of that effect is one of the most important steps you and your partner can take to stop it from happening. The first defense against heterosexual bed death is honesty. Being honest with your partner when you sense you're neglecting each other's physical desires is key. Getting offended is a bad sign. It means you're not fully engaged and that your ego is more important to you than the health of your relationship.

Another is not making time, but taking it. Grab time by the face and make it your bitch! It's your time. It doesn't rule you. You rule it. Stop saying you don't have time. You do. You just need to move the furniture around a little to make space for sex. Sure, it's work, but any marriage/partnership requires some of that. Those who don't think that's true are probably best suited to "confirmed singledom". If you're not willing to admit that your relationship has been forged between two fallible humans, you probably should go it alone. Denying that your sex life is waning, being egotistical about approaches from your partner to address it, or laziness about doing the work involved, are not going to help. These attitudes are going to lead to the revolving door.

I'm speaking from experience. That experience, while not the most fun part of my life with my beloved, has been formative and has made me a better partner, overall and certainly, a better sex partner. So how did that experience inform us both? How did we put a stop to protestations of there never being "enough time for sex", or of being "too tired"? Most importantly, how did we do it without blaming each other, or being hurtful? Here's what we did.

Making time your bitch

My love and I are both hardworking people. One important decision we have made in our lives was not to have children. That's not for everyone. I know. But it's a decision neither of us has ever regretted, so that factor has never been a question. But work and its demands, social obligations, family and all the myriad things in life that keep us busy can build up, exhaust people and push sex to the bottom of the list. It happened to us, about four years after we began co-habiting. That's not bad, as it's a generally accepted reality that most couples experience a diminishment in sexual intensity after the first two years together.

That's right. Only two years. So if any of our relationships are to last more than two years, it's highly advisable to that you take what I'm going to tell you next seriously.

At about the four-year mark, both my partner and I had continued with our careers, working hard as the General Manager of a large chain store (me) and the proprietor of a marketing consultancy (her). We were doing well, economically. We were prospering. But it was clear that focusing on our respective career paths had taken its toll. We were both tired. But more than just tired, we'd become so comfortable in each other's presence that weren't being as sensitive to one another as we'd been in the earliest layer of our relationship.

"I miss you," she said one day, over a hurried breakfast. We'd started to make a point of rising a little earlier in order to enjoy some time together in the early morning, regardless of how little of it there was.

"Me too," I replied, wistfully. We knew right then that we needed to act. My partner's tentative approach didn't lay blame. It didn't accuse. It was a simple statement of fact that got my attention. After about eight months of slow drift, with the television set numbing us into complacency, she had realized that someone needed to say something. One of us was always falling asleep in front of it – in our holey sweatpants, of course. Whoever remained awake would rouse the other before crawling off to bed – to sleep. We'd been using fatigue as an excuse to avoid the question of physical intimacy. But what was really in the way was the pacifying soporific effect of the TV.

So we turned it off for good. We loaded that sucker into the back of our SUV and drove it to the nearest Sally Ann. It was one of the best things we ever did for ourselves. Maybe some of you don't want to hear this, but that box is sucking the sexuality right out of your relationship. The time you spend staring at that thing is better spent with your partner. Some of that time is sex time. Interested now? I thought you might be.

Neilson, the company that monitors television viewing habits and derives ratings from them, conducted a study in 2014. This study revealed that the average American between the ages of 25 and 34 watches 27 and one half hours of television, each and every week. That's more than one *day*. But if you find that figure shocking, consider this – it goes up as we age. By the time we reach the 35 – 44 brackets, we're in for 33 hours and 40 minutes. After 45, the figure rises again to almost 44 hours per week.

That is one helluva lot of time. Some couples even watch television in different rooms, exacerbating the damaging effect this modern habit can have by adding physical isolation.

I'm going to assume that most of you are in the median group (35 – 44). Can we agree that you're still young and healthy (for the most part) and sexually robust? Can we agree you're still interested in regular sex with your partner, because you're reading this book? Then maybe it's time to kick your sex-undermining little friend out of the house, for good. We did it and we're glad. We spend our time on other things, now, including sex. Sex isn't just for Saturday night at our house (although it's part of the weekend fun). Because we have exiled the insidious influence of television from our home, we are healthier, more engaged with each and happier, all around. We have time, because we've made it our bitch by making one simple change in our lives.

Back to that "room mate" thing

OK. I know sweatpants are comfortable. The thing is that if they become your home uniform, then you have effectively "de-sexified" yourself. This is true whether you are a man or a woman. Throw those things away. I mean it. My love became a bit too attached to her pair of well-worn sweats. I got to the point at which I wondered if she had lost all her other clothes, except those she wore to work. So I asked her:

"Did something happen to your other clothes?"

"No," she answered, regarding me with wide, curious eyes. "Why are you asking me that?"

As gently as possible, I asked her where the silk lounging pajamas I'd brought her from the last convention I'd attended. I told her how sexy I thought she'd look in them and asked why she never wore them.

"Those are for special occasions, honey!" She giggled, coyly.

"Every day is a special occasion, where you're concerned." I said, smiling sweetly.

Without telling her she looked like a homeless person, or dumpy, I made it clear that the sweatpants were not doing it for me; that I wanted to enjoy her glory swaddled in something perhaps more enticing than those frigging sweats. I had planned for the occasion, thought about what I intended to say and how I intended to say it, beforehand. I'd also tidied up my own appearance, in preparation. Sauce. Goose. Gander. Women are visual, too, fellas. They like to see the man they originally fell in love with, occasionally.

Chapter 4: Every Day is a Special Occasion

Every day of your lives together is a special occasion. That's because it's another day of life for you both and none of us gets as many of those as we'd like. Best of all, you're living your lives *together*.

Recognizing every day as the gift it is reminds us that our time here is limited. Why waste it neglecting one of the best things in life there is? Seriously. That is no way to live. When my wife stopped wearing those sweatpants, it's not as though she put on crazy lingerie and pranced around for my entertainment (because that's for extra-special occasions). She just varied her home repertoire a bit to incorporate comfortable, eye-appealing loungewear. I did the same. In addition, when she came home from work, every day, she started to follow the ritual of removing her makeup and brushing out her hair (which is long and dark and threaded with grey). No one gets to see her that way, except me, her family and maybe a couple of very close friends. I like the intimacy of that gesture and she knows it.

Celebrating each other

Couples tend to save celebrations for those occasions they deem significant to them. With time, though, these can become few and far between. Even dinner out on Valentine's Day will seem like "waste", or "indulgence". But when it comes to celebrating your relationship and what each of you brings to it, it's important that you celebrate each other as often as possible and in unexpected ways that deepen your mutual appreciation and enhance the attraction that's still there and can be grown.

Random acts of kindness aren't just for people in the line up at the coffee shop, or grocery store. They're something the two of you should practice, bestowing some of that kindness on each other. Who should you be kinder to than the one who shares your life at the most intimate level possible? It's a no brainer.

Has she expressed an interest in something? Buy a book about it, throw that book in a gift bag and present it to her over the dinner you now have time to prepare together, post-TV. It doesn't have to be expensive. You can find books on virtually every subject possible at second hand stores which cost very little. Every gift, no matter how small, means you've been listening and taking note and thinking about each other.

Does he look particularly handsome in that tie? Tell him so. Then go out and pick him up a pocket puff to match it. Next time he wears the tie, tuck that sweet, thoughtful gesture into his jacket pocket before he leaves in the morning. Watch his face light up.

Offer to help each other with whatever needs to be done. That means housework, a project for work, or a problem with a friend or family. Be present to what your partner is saying and then respond with the hand you are in the relationship to offer when needed. It's part of living together.

Celebrating each other daily, in small ways, can be as simple as a text, an email, or a phone call. It doesn't have to be a dozen roses. It might be a special sandwich delivered to the office. It might be a call just to say that your love is on your mind. All these seemingly small things add up to a stronger bond between you. They show that you care. It doesn't matter how long you've been together, or how busy you think you are. You're never too busy to take a brief moment to check in. You're not being oppressive. You're being present.

Make a calendar of significant events in both your lives. These don't have to be events in your relationship. They can be events involving the family, like a birthday, or an anniversary. Celebrating the times that matter to each other is a sign of respect for your partner and for your partner's family. It demonstrates that you're engaged with the entire person you love the most, which means those your partner loves. You don't have to like them all. (That almost never happens, right?) What you should make a point of, though, is to know what matters to your partner and to honor it.

Chapter 5: Other Kinds of Foreplay

You've moved the furniture around to make space for your sex life. The TV is gone. The sweat pants – gone. You've both done some personal landscaping and maintained this practice as a hygiene discipline. You've both got a lot to give each other and we've discussed making sure you're reminding each other of that and celebrating it, on each special day of your lives together. Now all that's left is to get it on.

Knowing each other (in that Biblical sense and otherwise)

A lot of couples think they know each other, going in, only to find out in pretty short order just how little they know about each other. A lot of that knowledge has to do with sensitivity. As Marvin Gaye sang, "we're all sensitive people", whether we're tuned into that sensitivity or not. It's part of who we are. Learning about each other, because of this, is an emotional exploration of the way you both function, think and of course, express yourselves sexually.

What you know about each other sexually, if you've been together any length of time, is (no doubt) encyclopedic. Then again, if you're truly engaged lovers, you'll never stop learning and enjoying that education, as your lives together go on. You'll know when the time is right by a look, or a gesture. You'll know when it's not, too. The time isn't always right. Either one of you may be sick, or truly bagged. Both of you may just not be in that place at any given moment, or perhaps, only one of you. Like I've already said, mature people understand that libidos ebb and flow. It's all part of the joy of coupledom. This reality can be unpredictable, but honoring that ebb and flow is part of living out sexuality in a long-term relationship. You know when it's a naturally occurring state and when it's an indication you need to have an honest discussion. You know each other *that well* and knowing each other *that well* means that neither of you should feel inhibited about talking it out.

But when you're both ready, who initiates? Do you always wait for your partner to step up? Or do you take turns? Is there imbalance in this situation? You guessed it. My love and I have been through this one, too. She's usually the party with the plan. This is the case, because I sometimes bring work home with me. She does, too, but because of her organizational flair, she is much better able to put it in its place. Because of my lack of said organizational flair, I sometimes let working at home get the better of me – and of our sex life.

My partner had started to feel that I'd lost interest, during one arid spell we experienced, about ten years into our relationship. This wasn't the case, I made clear.

"Listen, baby. I can't help it if I have all this extra work," I put my hands on her waist, regarding her a little sheepishly. I knew what her answer to that was going to be.

"C'mon. You just need to be more organized!" She was right and so we embarked on an organizational project that was to revolutionize the way I worked at home, freeing my mind to wander to other, equally important matters. Of course, principle among those matters was occasionally surprising my wife by making an extravagant pass at her, when she least expected it. The change was great for me, for her and for us. All it took was a little life hack, courtesy of my hyper-organized partner.

I have to admit it was fun being in the driver's seat, for a change. She's pretty assertive!

Date night

If you've been reading carefully, you will know that I take romance pretty seriously. I believe in it and I know both men and women need it. Romance is the embroidery on a tablecloth. It's the strawberry in your champagne. The icing on your cake. Romance is the practice of making something beautiful more beautiful by taking a little extra care and deploying a little strategic planning. It pays off in so many ways.

Even if you've made more time in your life to keep the home fires lit, sometimes it's helpful to plan days and times you are going to promise one another a very special night. Invite your partner to the event. Say something sexy.

"I would be delighted to have the pleasure of your company for a bubble bath, followed by some extended nudity to the silken sounds of Marvin Gaye".

"Swoon!" will very likely be the response. This one is not gendered, folks. Men can invite women. Women can invite men. The idea of being invited to a special event gives you both something to look forward to. Pump up the volume with texts and emails: "Can't wait until tomorrow night." Or better yet, place a basket of bath products on the bathroom counter the morning of the planned festivities before your partner wakes up. Tuck a sexy note in there to drive the message home and crank up the anticipation factor.

Plan an evening out or take a walk in a romantic place. Maybe it's a local, urban park, or a riverside trail. Maybe it's dessert out, after dinner at home. Flirting over a piece of luscious cheesecake in a public place can be very titillating, especially if you're feeding it to each other. There are so many ways you can spend quality time together, even on a budget, that there's really no excuse. With the TV gone, put your time to good use by planning outings with each other that highlight your mutual interests and doing the things you both enjoy.

Play is for lovers

Adulting is tough. We're supposed to attend to the serious matters of adulthood, once we're grown and have flown the nest. Responsibility, having allegedly built our characters, now dominates our lives. Bills. Work. Responsibility. But being an adult doesn't mean we're supposed to stop having fun. Anyone who says it does should probably make a lateral move straight to the cemetery.

Fun and play are pleasures far too many of us push to one side, when we grow to adulthood. We claim not to have time for them. We think we're "too old" for them. We frown on those who continue to insist on having them in their lives. Arranging our sour pusses into the type of expression that says "some people never grow up", some of us turn up our noses at the antic behavior of these silly bastards.

Bravo, I say! Know why? Because I'm one of those silly bastards who will never grow up.

If there's a chance to dance, I am going to take it. Who knows how long I'll be able to? The day will come for all of us when we'll see people dancing and think "I'd give an arm for five more minutes on that dance floor". So why do we get ourselves tied up in knots about it? Who cares what anyone thinks? It's your life. It's yours to enjoy. Stop giving a damn.

Skinny-dipping is another favorite of mine. If there's water around and there's no one (who might be likely to arrest me) watching, I will run screaming like a banshee toward that water, shucking off my clothing as I go. My partner finds this endearing (thank God).

Fun and play are also key ingredients in my personal recipe for keeping relationships as fresh as a head of lettuce in the crisper. You and your partner need to play, have fun, tell each other jokes and get downright silly, sometimes. Take every opportunity you come across to let your inner wild child out to play. Doing that might give birth to some of the best memories you will ever share.

Youth is wasted on the young and bearing witness to that is a mandate! Believing you're too old to have fun (especially with your life partner) is a belief that kills more people than cancer, if you want my opinion. A life without fun, especially the kind of fun you can share with your lover, like dancing and skinny-dipping, or bowling, or parachuting from an airplane, or geo-caching, or throwing darts at the local pub, is not life. It's waiting for the Grim Reaper. Have the fun. Just do it.

Chapter 6: Let's Get it on – The Gospel According to Marvin Gaye

"We're all sensitive people
With so much to give
Understand me, sugar
Since we've got to be here
Let's live
I love you"
(Lyrics: Marvin Gaye/Ed Townsend)

Love is a many splendored thing, and a big part of its splendor is getting it on. Marvin Gaye is the prophet of this great truth and I strongly suggest that (if you haven't already) you make his sexual wisdom part of your life.

So turn on the stereo and let Marvin preach the gospel. Things are about to get mighty real.

Every time, the first time

Familiarity doesn't always breed contempt, but it can breed

the sort of romance-killing comfort that drives the "room mate" effect. You get so used to each other that you can't imagine a time when you weren't together. You finish each other's sentences. You finish each other's sandwiches. If you're not careful, you become siblings. Siblings are not lovers (one hopes).

So, if you're going to keep your sex life alive and kicking, you need to start with your eyes. Your eyes become so accustomed to seeing this person you know so well that they actually stop seeing them. Your image of that person transforms, over time, from blind infatuation (in which there is little, if anything, to fault) to a kind of bland, familial intimacy that is the exact opposite of passion. That starts with they way you look at each other; the way we interpret each other's presence.

Looking at your partner as though you were seeing that person for the very first time is about your attitude. Your sex life will improve, therefore, when your attitude toward your partner changes.

Look at your partner as though for the first time – and the last time. My mother used to say to me, when we were travelling places, "Take a good look. You don't know if you'll ever be back". She was right and this was some of the most solid (and poignant) advice I've ever been given. Later on in life, she confided that when my sister and I were small, she never wanted us to walk out the front door to go off to school on a sour note. She always made sure we left the house happy and feeling safe in her care. She said she did this because she couldn't be certain, from one day to the next, if we would meet again in this life. She was never very good at telling us she loved us, but this story makes it abundantly clear how much she actually did and continues to.

Life is uncertain and nothing is secure in it. Our illusions of security lull us into a false sense of life going on tomorrow the same as it does today. But this is never the case. Everything can change in a heartbeat. That's why your eyes need an upgrade. That's why you need to look at your partner as though seeing your love for the first time and the last.

Our physical appearances change, but these changes are the story of our lives. Couples share a story and so you need to look at your lover as a part of story you've been telling together. You are each other's historical romance. There is beauty to be seen in every line, every plane and every hollow of your faces and bodies. Reflect on this reality as you look at your partner. Shift your attitude about who you're looking at, setting aside cultural prejudices about what constitutes beauty. If you love your partner, then beauty is your partner.

Late one night, my love and I were driving home in the car from an event we'd attended at the home of friends. It was a hot night and the windows were open to the night air. She had her hand out the window, eyes closed and her feet up on the dash. I remember pulling up to a stop sign a few blocks from our place and looking over at her. She had fallen asleep and her head had fallen back. Her mouth was open. Just as I was thinking how stunningly beautiful she was, a rip-roaring snore came from her mouth. It was a sound I had difficulty believing this lovely creature could make and it surprised me so much, I started laughing and couldn't stop. Yet, she slept on. Not even the force of the snore could awaken her

Arriving home, I parked and went around to the passenger side to wake her up, but she was awake, looking up at me.

"What are you smiling about?" She blinked at me and yawned.

"You snore." I grinned. Her smile in return, a little dopey and glazed from sleep was even more beautiful than her sleeping face. And that night, I realized I was going to see her differently in the days and weeks and years to come, because I had seen something new in her that night and re-discovered the new depths of her wonder.

And that wonder is the foundation of our sex life. That wonder is what you need to hang on to. It's the miracle of loving someone and being alive, together, in the same moment in time. It's seeing a face for the first time and realizing you want to look at it for the rest of your life. Every day is the rest of your life and every day is both new and old. Seeing your partner as though for both the first time and the last time, is a gift which will inform your emotional approach to your partner and re-build it as a fresh reality, new and abundantly lovely.

Loving anew

The definition of insanity is doing the same thing over and over again and expecting different results. The same is true of sex. In fact, if the two of you keep doing the same thing over and over again, you'll soon find that you won't be doing it at all. Your playbook needs an overhaul.

The Greeks say you can't eat moussaka every day. Can you imagine eating the same food every day? Wearing the same clothes? How about that Bill Murray movie, *Ground Hog Day*? The guy's life was the same day, lived over and over again. How crazy would that drive you? Sex that isn't varied and surprising to you both isn't sex so much as it is something along the lines of trimming your toenails, or cleaning your belly button. You do it because you have to, not necessarily because it's fun. Routine is the sex killer. The same moves – sex killer. Boredom – sex killer. Don't let it happen. Learn to love anew.

That means paying attention to a number of different factors. Sit down and think about it. How does your love making sessions usually go? Do you generally conform to a certain pattern, in terms of initiation, foreplay (if there is any), sex positions and practices? Are you ever spontaneous about your love making, or do you routinely know approximately when it's going to happen, as though on a timer?

Think about the last time the two of your had sex. Think through it objectively, from start to finish. Now ask yourself if that's the best you can do. It's not. I'm willing to guarantee it. If you're reading this, I'm hoping it's because you genuinely want to regain the intensity you knew in the beginning of your relationship. It's possible, but it's going to take a little honesty on your part, as to how you can change your sexual behaviors and encourage your partner to change, with you. This isn't about pointing fingers, or "he said, she said". This is about stepping up and being completely honest with each other. But walking the talk is often the best way of sending the message.

Be the change you want to see in the bedroom. Free yourself from tired routines and both of your asses will follow. That's exactly what happened with us.

Slaying the sex killer dragon

You are a knight/knightess in shining armor, because you are now going to slay this dragon. Never will it lurk behind the laundry basket in the shadows of your bedroom again. No. You shall slay it with mighty blows and return bearing it's heading, having it separated it from its scaly body.

Slaying the sex killer dragon is a lot of fun. It's fun because you're going to become the lover your partner is going to fall in love with all over again. With your new eyes turned to "laser beam" and your new attitude, you're about to make loving fun again. Fun, playful and better than it has been for you and your partner for a while. What could be more fun than springing a few well-timed surprises? Everyone loves a surprise.

But remember – sexual dynamics can take time to shift. If you've been suffering from heterosexual bed death, then somebody needs to make a move, but move with caution. Rushing up on this shift can result in trauma. Women readers shouldn't suddenly appear at the side of bed with what amounts to a threat to strapped to your body. If there are sex practices you'd like to try, but that may be beyond the scope of either of your experience, it always pays to bring it up before throwing yourself at your lover, nipple clamps first. So talk is where it all begins.

You don't need to sit your partner down for a "talk". You need, rather, to set your partner up for what's to come. That means being increasingly present in your affections, your attentions and your approach. A touch here, a kiss there, wrapped in a whispered suggestion can signal that a new era has dawned in your lives together. It sends the warm message that life is about to get a lot more fun and a lot sexier.

Crank up the Marvin Gaye, arch your eyebrow just the right way and get ready to take your partner on the ride of a lifetime. Ladies and gentlemen, start your engines.

Chapter 7: Foreplay as Erotic Overture

In the world of opera, as some readers will know, the overture is what's played before the main event starts. This piece of music sets the scene for what the audience is going to hear and see over the course of the entertainment. If opera is one of the great musical art forms, sex is a physical counterpart. Like opera, sex is a discreetly blended balance of emotion, magic, artistry and story telling. Yes. Story telling. You're writing love on each other's bodies and your love is a story with many scenes, unfolding as you express the meaning of that love physically.

So foreplay isn't optional. It's part and parcel of sex. Foreplay is especially necessary for women and that means it's important that men become proficient in what works for their women in terms of foreplay and work to expand their repertoire in order to give women what they need.

Sometimes, foreplay is more limited (quickies – which are piles of fun, in a pinch). Sometimes, it's extended, languid and lingered over. Sometimes it's something else entirely (banter, teasing, secret caresses). As with all sex, the threat of the sex killer dragon looms ever near the peripheries of your foreplay game. Just because you've cut off one sex killer dragon's head doesn't mean to say another isn't going to take its place. That can happen in your foreplay, too. Relying too heavily on one thing or another, not talking to your partner, not being present to your partner's responses, or being too intent on getting to the main course, can impact how good it is for both of you.

Getting the ball rolling

Being tentative and ambiguous about being in the mood for love is no way to get the ball rolling. The ball is not going to roll, for example, if you ask your partner, "Do you feel like having sex right now?" Captain Obvious, please. There is nothing sexy about that. You're not asking if your lover feels like sharing a sandwich. You're asking if your lover feels like getting naked with you and enjoying each other's bodies.

That means taking an entirely different approach. Words can be so limiting. Touch and gaze can be more eloquent ways of sending the message that you're ready for love. A nose nuzzling an earlobe, or a finger tracing the curve of the cheek speak volumes. Men are particularly susceptible to falling into bed with their partners by way of a well-placed touch. When a man's partner, for example, places her hands on his chest, her fingers perhaps straying to the top button, suggestively, as she looks up at him through her eyelashes, she will enjoy almost immediate results. Women are always fond of being approached in this way, but with gentle consideration to their different way of interpreting sexual signals. Men should be aware of the way their touch speaks to women, as the history of womanhood is marred by male violence. It doesn't matter if you're one of the rotten scoundrels who treat our beloved sisters in this way. Women pick up on things. Be aware of what your hands are saying, as you place them on her rounded hips. Whisper what you're thinking in her ear, as you do it and there will be no question.

The ball can get rolling long before either of you gets anywhere near the bedroom. First thing in the morning, over breakfast, at lunch, or during a brief call in the middle of the afternoon. A suggestive email or text message are new ways of fanning the flames that you'll want to take full advantage of. Using all these forms of communication, in combination, can build the right kind of tension between the two of you. That lustful, anticipatory vibe is what you're looking for.

Sexual flirting in public is also a lot of fun. My partner and I do this all the time. Our friends know when we're doing it, as we've been doing it for so long and so publicly (because we don't care what anyone thinks of it). They bug us about it. That's part of the fun. We take pride in being the most libidinous couple in our social circle and you will, too.

We spend most Christmases in the bosom of my love's family. Christmas, in the midst of this large, somewhat unhinged and resolutely Anglo-Irish family, is the usual procession of sugar cookies, teething babies, endless food and ample booze going down the neck of our obligatory drunk uncle. Family is a wonder and Christmas, in her family, is one of the great wonders of the world. There is loud singing and often, dancing. There's usually some sort of altercation (which unfolds almost like a bad episode of performance art). We take it all in with a smile of grateful, slightly buzzed happiness and carry on as we always do, engaged in building the sexual tension between us. Then, once we're good and cranked up and the relatives are bellowing about the outrage of the day, we'll kick it into high gear.

"I think I need nap." She'll say, quietly, as the drunken uncle expounds on the evils of capitalism and store bought beer.

"Mmm. (Yawn). Me too." I will stretch as extravagantly as a cat, reaching for the ceiling, dramatically and unmistakably fatigued.

And so, as the family rages, locked in its traditional squabbles over the world's ills, we slip away, up the stairs to a quiet room, and do what we do best. For years, we believed we'd pulled off our annual caper without detection. The smug, private leers we shared over the familial turkey, our lingering afterglow. But this past Christmas, we looked up from one such shared leer to see our now righteously drunk uncle leering back. With a pull on his whiskey and a lascivious wink, he burst our bubble. Surely if he knew, they all must.

But it's all in the family and if they all know, then it's now a Christmas tradition. It can be your Christmas, or Passover, or Thanksgiving tradition, too. For us, it's one of the shared behaviors that keep our life as a loving couple rosy with fresh life. I highly recommend Holiday quickies at the family get together, for this reason.

I want to close this section by making one important point — telling your partner they're attractive and that they turn you on, is one of the best ways to get the ball rolling and keep it rolling it as a daily habit. I make a point of complimenting my lover. Sometimes it's what she's wearing. Sometimes it's a new scent. Sometimes, it's the way a pair of jeans is clinging to her rear end. Men may believe they're above this sort of appreciation, but that's nonsense. We need to feel sexually attractive, too. That's why some of us buy a sports car in mid-life. It makes us feel desirable to the opposite sex. It makes us believe that someone, somewhere is paying attention to little old us and you bet we need attention. Any man who says otherwise isn't being honest with himself.

Express your appreciation of each other regularly. Be specific. Does he look hot in that suit? Tell him. Tell him you like his Saturday morning stubble on the back of your neck. Tell her she's as beautiful without her makeup on as she is with it. Be each other's biggest fans. There's nothing sexier.

The approach

I have a friend who swears up and down that jumping out of a closet naked is the best possible way to signal to his partner that it's time for love. Many a tale he's shared of the success of this strategy, so adamant is he that it works like a charm. It works for him. I tried it. It did not work for me. I scared the crap out of my partner and she refused to speak to me for the rest of the evening (much less, do anything else with me). You can try it. Just keep in mind that results have not been verified by any sample larger than my friend and me. That's a 50% chance, which is not that great, if you ask me.

Personally, I think there are much better ways of approaching one's lover, if you've put a little time and thought into building the sexual tension between the two of you. Romance is the key to this. That doesn't have to mean production numbers of Cecil B. DeMille proportions, but it does mean that you must employ your masculine/feminine wiles to the good.

Wiring is for computers

Every time I hear or read about men and women being "wired" differently, I cringe a little. I cringe a little because I know I'm not a robot and I know my partner isn't a robot, either. We're human beings. We are not composed of wires and circuitry. We're not binary creatures. And by the way, we're not all the same, regardless of which side of the (perceived) divide we're on. Human beings are vastly and wildly varied animals, with hugely diverse backgrounds that include genetics, experience and all manner of information stuffed into our high-functioning brains.

Once again, we need to know our partners to really get to the bottom of what turns them on. That means keeping the lines of communication open. But it also means understanding that there are some fairly reliable differences between men and women we should talk about.

There's a picture floating around the interwebs that depicts the difference between men and women in terms of circuitry. A machine with a bunch of switches is shown on the top half of the picture. Wires snake out from it in every direction. It's a complicated-looking thing. On the lower half of the picture, a machine with a single button is shown. Guess which is intended to depict how males "work".

Personally, I find it more than a little depressing that

someone out there (probably a man, as some of us tend to take pride in the "simple creatures" construct) has reduced me to a push button appliance. I am not that simple. I'm sure men reading this will agree that they're not all that "simple" either. I have more than one button. I have more than one switch. And like I said, I'm not a machine, or a robot. I'm a flesh-and-blood creature with all the attendant bells, whistles and quirks and I'm proud of it.

The fundamental difference between men and women is a little subtler. Some of that difference is found in our brains and their chemical realities, but most of this difference is culturally driven. Women have been conditioned to respond in certain ways and so, require something a little more than wink, a nod and bra flung unceremoniously on the kitchen floor, to signal they'd like to get it on. Women need to feel desired. Men need that too. Don't get me wrong. But women demand just a little more emotional appeal and there's something men can learn from that, in terms of finding the sexual sweet spot with their partners. So let's look at some approaches for men to employ, when wooing their partners (and wooing is something which should be continued for the life of the relationship) into bed.

Come hither, fair maiden – for men

Here's a thought to consider – a lot of men tend not to touch their partners with any affection unless they're approaching them for sex. My partner regales me with pseudonymous, second hand stories from the annals of the sex lives of her friends with their respective partners. For the most part, these tales are sad. When partners feel disconnected from each other, or when one feels neglected, the outcome is never pretty. That's why it's so important for both men and women to continue to "see" each other and equally importantly, to "feel" each other.

Something I've learned about my love over the years is that she needs to hear from me that's she's sexy. She needs to know that I feel turned on by being near her and that I'm proud and happy to be with her. My habit of making sure that's the case, which is now part of our daily lives, has drawn us closer together as a couple. And that is key to the approach. That emotional closeness makes drawing together physically so much easier.

Once established, the approach of a man to his woman partner becomes a delicious dance of communicative foreplay. Don't make her guess. Make her understand. You can start this dance wherever you are, by establishing that the time is right. What's she doing later? What does she feel like doing? Are there any lose threads in her day that may need to be attended to? Don't just assume she's available. That assumption is the kiss of certain death. Too many romantic partnerships assume that both partners are light switches (there's that "wiring" thing again), capable of being turned on at will. But life isn't like that.

So your job, first and foremost, is to establish that she's down. Once that's out of the way, you can begin your inexorable, romantic approach. Much of this depends on establishing a mood of impending sex, by inciting her lust. If there's cologne you know she likes, be wearing it. Maybe go take a shower and emerge in those boxers she likes to see you in. You might want to sit down in front of her as you dry your hair, smiling at her boyishly, all the while.

But whatever it is you do, remember that you're *approaching*. Your woman is not an objective. She's your other half. You're reaching out for *that*. You're not grabbing a body part, or cheerfully bellowing that you're in the mood for love. A man who knows his partner doesn't have to do that. A man who knows his partner is aware of her sexual triggers and how he might gently activate them, until the moment of arousal has arrived. Desire and arousal are two different animals. Women tend to feel desire long before arousal arrives, whereas men experience them almost simultaneously, for the most part. That's important to remember. While she may be in a state of desire, she needs you to trigger her to get to arousal. Know her triggers, whether they're cologne, boxers, briefs, Marvin Gaye, or scented oil in a pretty burner on the coffee table. Even poetry may be a sexual trigger for a woman. Just know.

Hey stud – for women

Despite what we say, men need to know we're sexy and that women into us as much as women need to know their men are into them. We need to feel desired and "manly". We need to feel as though your knees go weak at the sight of us.

Men also like visuals, so your knowledge of your male partner's triggers in that department (lingerie, to example) is important. Some men are turned on by woman removing her makeup and presenting a fresh face to him and him alone (especially if she's highly groomed in her daily life). For such men, your message to him is one of exclusivity, which is a way of reassuring him that your love is a private affair, to be shared between only the two of you. While some men enjoy the sight of their women in lacy lingerie (suddenly revealed in a dramatic way, perhaps, like a dress dropping to the kitchen floor), others are triggered by something different. That can be anything from one of his t-shirts over your underwear, or even a housecoat (with nothing underneath it).

A lot of men enjoy women taking the lead, but as with every other rule of thumb, that's not a global rule. Some men are taken aback by feminine sexual aggression and can completely turn off when they encounter it. As I told you earlier, that's certainly not the case with me. In fact, my partner even had to point out that it would be nice if I could initiate sometimes, so I do that, now. She's still the boss, though! Still, understanding your man and how he responds to you making the initial come on is an important factor. Play with it. Switch your game up. If that means appearing at his side nude, as he sits at the computer, what the heck! Men are just as complicated as women, when it gets down to it. Some things work better than others and some things don't work well at all.

And just like women, every moment is not going to be the right moment. When he's in the middle of a difficult episode at work, or with his family, don't expect him to shift gears any faster than you do. All systems are not going to be "go" all the time. That's just the way life is and men are just as vulnerable to that reality as women are. I know this runs counter to popular sexual mythology, but everything in life (especially your sex life) can't be boiled down to a stereotype. That may be one of the most important messages of this book.

Chapter 8: Fresh Horses for Longtime Lovers

One of the best things you and your partner can do for each other is to play a little game my lover and I enjoy often. We take a little time each week to search for new ideas to spring on the other. We review all incoming information through the filter of our knowledge of each other.

"But will it play in Peoria?" This should be the first question you ask about any planned introduction of a new move into your sexual repertoire. There's plenty out there to choose from, to be sure. That doesn't mean all of it's for you, or that revisions aren't in order. All advice on the market concerning bringing some additional dazzle to your already dazzling line up of stock moves, is subject to your critical gaze.

Customization is a good word to describe what happens to some of this advice when incorporated into our lovemaking routine. If we try something (and like it), it stays. That doesn't mean we're going to roll it out each and every time we get it on. It means it's hanging in the closet, like a favourite shirt, tie or blouse. It's ready to be put on again. Not necessarily tomorrow, or even next week. But we know it's there.

Beyond Missionary

We all have our "go to" moves in the bedroom. But how long does it take for "go to" to become "go home"? Not long, boys and girls. Let's face it, there's nothing more tedious than being able to anticipate, with way too much accuracy, how your sexual encounters are going to unfold.

"Well, first – this will happen and then, this, closely followed by that. The end."

That does not sound exciting to me. Does it sound exciting to you? I doubt it. So how do you break what amount to bad habits in the bedroom and give your sex life the boost it needs to bring it back to vibrant life?

Spin the wheel. In this and the following chapters, I'm going to give you a little reference guide to some of the more fun and interesting sex positions and practices out there. This is just a small sampling of ways you and your lover can renovate your sex life, to make it more varied and fun and to get out of the rut too many couples get into after that initial love-madness wears off.

As you read, I hope you'll get a little tingle from what's on offer here. I also hope you'll be creative about how you intend to introduce this advice into your playtime repertoire. There's no need to take an ad out in the paper. You can have fun with this too, dropping hints about "having something special for later on". Encourage your partner to do the same, either with this book, or with other resources. The idea is to please, delight and surprise each other with the new goodies you're bringing to your sex life. These are gifts of love and consideration for each other's pleasure and yet another way to show each other how very alive your love truly is.

Some of what we're going to review in the pages that follow are:

- Sex positions you may have wanted to try, but were too shy to.

- Sex positions to encourage and enhance female orgasm

- Helpful tips to delay male orgasm (see above)

- Oral sex

- Manual sex

- Sex aids and helpers

- Furnishings

- Sex positions for those with physical limitations (older readers, disabled and post-surgical suggestions). Just because nobody seems to pay a lot of attention to you folks.

- Other types of sex play which you may have wanted to try, but were too shy to.

Note that I've left the more adventurous item for the end. We're going to work up to that bit, as I realize that this may be the very first time some of you have read a book like this. I'm going to ease you into it (just the way we're learning to ease into sex, as me might a nice, hot bath). You're learning to be more open and honest about your sexual desires with your partner and trying new things is part of that openness and honesty. It's a process and I understand that, because I've been through it with my lover. There's nothing to be shy about. Sex is supposed to be fun and it's way more fun when you're both on the same page and ready to spread your wings and fly to lands unseen.

And now, we're ready to open up the vault and pull out some new tricks, moves and toys to make everyone's sex lives just a little more fun, playful and varied.

Chapter 9: Sex Positions You May Have Wanted to Try but Were Too Shy to

I'm sure some of you use lubrication (other than what occurs naturally) in your sex play, but additional lubrication is always advised. Why? Because it's a peripheral. Because it's not naturally occurring, there's something about it that seems almost naughty. It also *feels* naughty, due to the additional slipperiness it provides. Lubrication also provides us with enhanced stamina, due to the reduction of the friction that can occur when sex is prolonged. It pays to use it and so I suggest you make room for it in your sex life, before introducing anything described in this book into your sex play. I'll cover the various types of lube in a later chapter. For now, though, plan on adding it to your sexy time shopping list.

We've probably all had sex in the standard variation of this position, but there are a couple of tweaks here that make that standard model a little more special.

The clamp

This is an "off road" position, in that it's performed on the side of the bed. The woman kneels next to the bed's edge, with her upper body across it, supported on her hands, knees together. The man stands behind her, with feet hips width apart.

Because the woman's knees are together, the entry is to be achieved slowly and carefully and with the help of lubrication. Once in, men will note how different this variation of the "doggy style" position is from the one they're used to. The effect is that of a clamp and this can be heightened by the woman's use of the pelvic floor muscles, to grip the man's penis, as sex proceeds.

If you're reading carefully and thoughtfully, you'll understand that this position isn't one to start with. It's pretty intense and it's likely a lot of men won't be able to last long (especially if their women have been doing their Kegel exercises regularly).

Standing Beast

This one is particularly good for when the mood strikes you at an inopportune time and there just happens to be a friendly and convenient closet, bathroom, or otherwise out-of-the-way corner, wherever you're at, to avail yourselves of.

With the woman's back against the wall and her legs wrapped around the man, this one demands a little strength and balance, but is well worth the effort. Don't worry about not having the stamina to make it work. Neither of you will need it, if the mood has struck you with such force in a public place, that you're about to get it on against the most convenient wall (Marvin Gaye, or no). If the space is particularly small, even better, as the woman can use the opposite wall to brace her feet against and help with the heavy lifting. That's why I particularly like closets for this position.

Squatting Cowgirl

Most of us have enjoyed the "backward cowgirl" at some point, in which the woman mounts the man, with her back to him. This variation is very similar, but with a decided twist. The woman squats in front of the man, between his open legs, which should be bent at the knee. Supporting herself by placing her hands on his knees, she then mounts him, with her back to him. She controls the action by using his knees for leverage.

Once again, the woman's knees being in the position they are can make for added intensity, so it's advisable that this one be left for later stage lovemaking. Lubrication is strongly advised.

Crabwalk

Remember when you were a kid in school and this was one of the races you did at sports day? Remember the tall, skinny kid who couldn't walk in a straight line, but invariably won this race; his freakishly long limbs propelling him to crabwalk dominance, each and every year?

You've got the picture.

You're facing each other, both in this position. The woman's legs go on either side of the man's body. Both partners are supporting themselves on their hands. This means that both can participate in the thrusting action. Once you're lined up properly, it's not half as complicated as it sounds and very exciting, for a needed change of pace.

Backwards Missionary

All missionary position sex isn't bad, but we'll get there shortly. It's just too pedestrian to be practiced incessantly. Everyone needs a little variety in their lives, because the Greeks were absolutely right about eating moussaka ever day. No. One cannot. Therefore, here's an interesting twist on the missionary position.

The woman assumes the position usually assumed for standard missionary. The man, alternatively, lies with his head over her feet. Where's the lube! You're going to need it for this one. Entry is achieved with the penis facing down from its accustomed, erect position. The woman can use her hands on her man's buttocks to help guide the action. Proceed with caution and the knowledge that penises need to get used to this manoeuver.

Bouncy, Bouncy

If you don't have an exercise ball in your home, then you may want to obtain one. These little items are good for a lot more than exercise and I'm about to tell you why.

This is another variation on the "reverse cowgirl", but with a bouncy, exercise ball twist. The man is seated on the ball. The woman, her back to the man, sits down on him. Her legs may be either open (outside his thighs), or closed (inside his thighs). The closed option, like others that involve this position of the woman's leg, will require adequate lubrication. Make sure the exercise ball has sufficient air in it to give a nice, bouncy ride and take care to stay on the ball!

X-tra Control

This position is a little bit missionary and a little bit reverse cowgirl, but much less frenetic and active. This move gives the woman a lot of control, as well, as she controls the depth of penetration and speed and intensity of thrusting.

With the man lying on his back, the woman lies on top of him, her head over his feet. Her legs should extend up either side of his body, her feet over his shoulders. Entry can be achieved from almost the "normal" erect position, with the woman pulling the penis downward, as she lowers herself between the man's legs. From here, she can hang on to his lower legs to provide leverage for thrusting, sliding up and down. Again, keep the lubrication near for maximum enjoyment.

Tight and High

In this one, the man takes the wheel, with the woman lying facing down and legs together. Her hips should be slightly raised for better access and maximum enjoyment. Use a pillow. There are plenty of specially designed pillows on the market, just for sex (like the wedge, which is described in the chapter on sex toys). Part of the fun of this position is that the man can gently massage the woman as she lies there anticipating penetration. Warm massage oil is always good for this.

When the moment's right, gentlemen, lube up and off you go.

Side Saddle

In the most ladylike way possible, the woman partner sits on the edge of the bed (or any other amenable piece of furniture, really), with her thighs together. She then leans on her forearm and one thigh, with the male partner entering from behind. As with all the "tight" entry positions describe herein, lubrication is helpful. But this position backs a punch, especially for women with superior control of pelvic floor muscles, so you may want to reserve this one for the grand finale!

Better Missionary

The missionary position gets a bad rap. But it's a "go to" for good reason. The intimacy of this time-honored sex position is undeniable, as it allows for the kind of face-to-face connection many couples prefer. Women especially like it for this reason. While it shouldn't dominate your sex play, it's one of my favorites, because it allows partners to see each other's eyes and faces and connect with each other in that old-fashioned way.

But there are ways to make this position even better.

Skin-to-skin contact in this position is maximized and that's a very good thing. There's nothing like the feeling of your skin pressed against that of your lover. Pump up the volume by making use of your hands and being aware of the sensations arising from the contact your bodies are making. Heighten your sensitivity to this physical contact by retreating from it (if you're the man and on top) from time to time. Hover over your woman and then zoom back in, with a passionate kiss. Roll around and lay side to side. Now roll to the other side. Move your hands over your lover's body, as you whisper in each other's ears. Tell each other what your hands are feeling. Feed each other's lust.

Women can also change the position of their legs to intensify their involvement, when in the missionary position. Part of the problem is that missionary is a "male dominant" sex position, that implicitly demands a certain sexual passivity from the woman. This can be remedied by a simple change in leg position.

A woman planting her feet on the bed, or one foot, can change the game completely. Men can also improve the effect of this position by ensuring that they're up on one elbow and hovering slightly. This allows an enhanced ability, on the part of the woman to move her hips in rhythm with her partner's.

Placing the woman's legs along the length of the male partner's body can also be intensely pleasurable for women. With her feet next to the man's ears, there is a slightly increased physical demand on him, but it's well worth the effort. Men can hang on to their women's ankles, while the woman's hands are free to roam. The deep penetration allowed in this variation on the traditional missionary will be highly pleasing to both partners.

Chapter 10: Sex Positions to Encourage and Enhance Female Orgasm

Sex is a two-way street. I'm of the very firm opinion that men who either don't care enough about their women's orgasms to make sure they have them (each and every time), or just don't care whether their women have them are not, don't really deserve to be with women at all.

You heard me. You don't deserve them.

At lot of women will swear up and down that it doesn't really matter. It's not that big a deal if you get yours and they don't get theirs. They're lying. But before you get your y-fronts in a twist, male readers, you should know that you are the reason they lie about it.

Women lie about it being just fine with them that they don't get to enjoy the "Big O" every time we have sex with them, because you are so defensive about your performance and sensitive about your manhood that they fear bruising you. They fear you'll be hurt and upset and dissolve into a puddle before their very eyes if they tell you that they expect you to make more of an effort when it comes to making sure they're satisfied.

Sometimes, women find a way to avoid the discussion altogether, though. That's when they tell another, more harmful lie. They tell you that they've had an orgasm when they haven't had one. They fear that if they tell you they haven't had an orgasm that you will fall to little bitty pieces right before their very eyes.

And why is that fellas? If the foregoing describes you in any way, then you know why. You know that you're a little delicate when it comes to sexy times and your virility. You don't want to hear that you're not the conquering hero, bearing sexual satisfaction wherever you go, because you are "the man". But the problem is that you will never be "the man", if your woman is not enjoying at least one orgasm each and every time you have sex.

Real men make sure their women come. You have time to help get her there, if you have time to have sex. If you think you don't, then guess what? You're not even having sex. You're masturbating with a woman present.

Yuck right? Right. Yuck.

I'm including these positions as silver bullets to your female partner's orgasm. But this chapter isn't the end of it. After this one, you're also going to learn how to delay your own orgasm for the sake of hers. That's what real men do.

Good Old Mr. Pillow

A nice, fluffy, springy pillow can be your best friend in the bedroom and can enhance your woman's ability to orgasm. Whether you're in the missionary position or entering from behind, elevating the woman partner's hips to facilitate entry and vary the angle of entry is one very effective way of increasing her arousal and thus, her ability to orgasm. Lubrication to intensify the pleasure is also highly advisable, especially when you're using that lubrication to encourage her to manually stimulate herself while you're having intercourse, or if you're doing that on her behalf. Good Old Mr. Pillow can be your very best friend. (Read about purpose-built sex pillows in the chapter on sex furniture).

The Spoon

Most of us know this one's not just for sleeping and/or cuddling. The Spoon can also encourage the female partner's orgasm. With your partner lying on her side in front of you, you spoon up to her from behind. This position doesn't allow full penetration, so (depending on the angle, which can be changed with slight adjustments to both your bodies' positions), you will be able to stimulate your partner's G-spot. The spoon can also be tweaked to involve the woman lying partially face down, with one leg bent. This variation allows somewhat greater penetration, but will still allow you to vary the depth and angle, according to your partner's responses (which you should be paying close attention to).

Your penis should not be thrust in more than 1 and ½ inches to 2 inches and should be pressed against the front wall of her vagina. Slow and regular thrusts are what you need to make this position result in what your partner needs from you – an orgasm achieved vaginally. You can also encourage your partner to squeeze you as you thrust in an out, which will further enhance both your pleasure.

The Chair

You can do this one just about anywhere, even on the side of the bed. I suggest, though, that you use a freestanding chair. A kitchen chair is perfect for this one. With the man seated, the woman partner turns her back and sits down. Her legs are together, while his are open. She can use her hands to push herself up and down on his thighs (or on the arms of the chair, if there are any). The woman, in this position, is free as a bird to explore the various angles and depths of penetration possible, which are numerous. She can even lean forward, with the man hanging on to her waist to create quite a bombastic effect for both parties involved. This is one of my partner's all time favorites and one we frequently enjoy. Pull up a chair and enjoy!

Catbird Seat

This one may sound a little complicated to you at first, but believe me, it's also really effective, if your goal is to make sure the woman you love is getting what she needs. Your partner is in charge again (so enjoy that). She will be on her knees, with one knee between your legs and the other, at your side. Bend one leg and plant your foot on the bed. Your partner will then guide your penis into her, using your bent leg as support. The angle of your penis and the friction provided by this position may demand the use of lubrication, so keep it handy.

Of all the positions my partner and I employ to bring her to the ultimate pleasure offered by human sexuality, these are the ones we've found to be most effective. A little later on we'll talk about some other sexual methods you can use to achieve the same effect, if you'd rather your partner get there before you do, or for her first orgasmic event of the night (as more than one is always preferred, if you're man enough). Remember, sex is a two-way street and her orgasm is just as important and just as crucial to the endeavor as yours. Without it, you really haven't had sex at all.

Chapter 11: Helpful Tips to Delay Male Orgasm

Now that we've talked about the importance of female orgasm in the grand scheme of your sex life, let's talk about some ways that you men can delay orgasm. This is not something you're going to need to do each and every time. But one thing's certain, enhancing your staying power is going to help you get more out of sex, yourself. This isn't just about making your partner happy. Every sexual occasion isn't intended to be a "quickie". Unfortunately, the male drive to orgasm can be a powerful thing and sometimes, we just roll with it. That's a mistake. When we give in to that, we're denying ourselves the full range of pleasure available to us in the unitive sex act. This is especially true of the sex we have in our long-term partnerships.

Being with our partners over a long period of time should be seen as invitation to ingenuity and imagination. Too often, though, our long-term relationships are seen as more of an invitation to the laziness engendered by comfort and familiarity. But did you know that women find that even more boring than men do? If some of you are reading this because you're fed up with your woman partners "having a headache", maybe you need to ask yourself if you're not the source of the pain?

If you're rolling on and then rolling off, only to fall into a deep and snoring sleep, then yeah, sorry. It's you. It's not her. You need to be the lover she fell in love with, just as she needs to be that for you. That means not giving in to laziness, because laziness is the same as taking her for granted and that can spell big trouble in your sex life and in your relationship as a whole.

Also, it's important for all men to get over the idea that orgasm is the sexual goal. Sex is about a lot more than orgasm. It's about you, as a whole person, relating to your woman as a whole person. You are whole people and your sexuality is a total physical expression. It's not a series of motions you go through to get what you really came for. We all love orgasms (love, love, love), but focusing on the destination can get in the way of the journey and that's where you really connect with your partner, on the deepest level. If you're so interested in your orgasm that you're rushing through your sex play to get there, then you may as well be in the bathroom with a magazine. Crude? So is being an inconsiderate, lousy lover.

So here are some tips to get a handle on your staying power and to make sure you're not heading yourself off at the pass, right before the good stuff gets rolling.

The perineum

Some of you may know this as the "gooch", or the "landing

strip". This is the little stretch of man located behind the scrotum and just in front of the anus. This little guy can be a tremendous help when you're seeking to delay your orgasm for the sake of quality sex and your female partner's orgasm.

This little trick has been in use by practitioners of Kama Sutra, Tantra and Taoism for centuries. By locating it and pressing on it when the urge to ejaculate arises, you can delay and even stop ejaculation. In truth, ejaculation is the result of orgasm. Orgasm is actually occurring before ejaculation and I guess we all know that, so that's the point at which we need to employ this tactic.

By pressing upward into the perineum (up to about the first knuckle), we can stop ourselves from letting loose and raining on our partners' parades (quite literally). But there's another trick you can use in conjunction with this one to make it even more powerful.

How to flex your pubococcygeus (PC) muscles

Those of you who go to the gym probably don't know how to flex these particular muscles, but they're way more important, in terms of sex, than your biceps, so let's find out more about them.

We've all heard of Kegel exercises. These enhance the strength of the muscles of the pelvic floor, for women. Sometimes these can be weakened by childbirth, or just age (like all our other human muscles), which can lead to incontinence, which is no fun at all. Kegel exercises can restore these muscles to their former strength, which can have some pretty amazing sexual benefits for the women who do them and the men they love. Locating the muscles in question by stopping the flow of urine while urinating, women can learn to exercise and strengthen these muscles. Let's find out how to do that with the male PC muscles.

You can find your PCs the same way women can find their Kegels. Go to the bathroom and begin urinating. Now, stop the flow. Take note of the muscles employed. Do this more than once, if necessary. Once you can do this with ease and feel confident about what happens when you stop the flow of your urine, you are in command of your PCs.

Now that you know where they are, you'll want to do some repetitions. Twenty of these, done three times daily and held for two seconds each, will soon have made you a PC master. Add ten slow squeezes when you feel ready, holding for a count of five and releasing slowly for five counts. This level of control is what you're after. Add the ten slow squeezes to your three rapid squeeze sets, each day.

There's an advanced version of the PC squeeze that a lot of you will get a bit of a thrill from. I certainly do. Do the same exercises, with an erect penis! What could be more fun? Throw a washcloth over your erection and practice raising it by squeezing your PCs. You are now not only a PC master, but can amuse your ladylove with your new skill, just for the giggles (and yes, she will giggle – every time).

Being a PC master means that when you want to interrupt ejaculation by pressing on your perineum, you can also employ your PCs to make the effect even more pronounced, thus increasing your ability to withhold ejaculation until you've reached a more opportune moment in the festivities. That means more fun for both of you and that should be your goal. Orgasm is a wonderful thing, but when you're staring, with single-minded focus at that one tree, a whole forest is passing you by. Keep that in mind and keep the party going.

Chapter 12: Oral Sex

Oral sex is a favorite for a lot of people and its wonder is that you can get away with doing it in a lot of different places (including the car, even if one of you is actually driving – but don't tell anyone I told you that).

For men, oral sex is a highly-beloved activity, so women need to pay some particular attention to this activity and how it's done right. While many women may believe that they're particularly good at this and while their men may lovingly tell them that's the truth, it's not always true. As with the female orgasm and the innocent lies women tell about it, sometimes men will lie to protect the feelings of their lovers. But let's face it, good "head" is a rather important component of sex for a lot of men, so women should be ready, willing and able not only to do it well, but also to enjoy it.

And therein lies the rub. Some women have a real problem with this one and that's a problem for their partners. Let's keep in mind here, that (as I've said earlier) sex is a two-way street and everyone on that street has an equal right to enjoy him or herself to the fullest. Oral sex is on the sexual menu, so if you're a woman who doesn't enjoy it, perhaps it's time to start thinking about why that is.

Some women have a history that has caused them to have a less than healthy relationship with oral sex. Others have hygiene concerns. Still others have a highly active gag reflex that's triggered by oral sex. Sometimes that's psychological, but sometimes there's a physiological response that's really the result of a psychological trigger. There's no woman in the world, though, who's Linda Lovelace. (In the film, Deep Throat, she plays a woman with a clitoris in her throat). Everyone reading this knows that's physiologically impossible.

But you don't need to have a clitoris in your throat to enjoy fellatio (oral sex performed on a man). Let's talk a walk through some thoughts on how to improve you/your partner's attitude with respect to going "downtown". The first section is about fellatio, but men shouldn't believe, for one second, they're getting off the hook. Women need you to go downtown too, so we're going there.

Avoiding the gag reflex

Being nervous about performing fellatio can actually make the gag reflex worse than it already is. So the key is for women to slow down their approach, stop thinking about how well they are or are not doing and to breathe. Breathing is key to relaxation and a lot of giving successful head has to do with exactly that. Being relaxed is most important part.

It's not necessary for good oral sex to be an athletic feat. It does not all have to go in your mouth at the same time, women readers. In fact, it's much more exciting for a man, if you employ multiple techniques that involve exactly the opposite. Shifting the intensity of the action and building it up is a turn on for men, but the biggest turn on of all is to see that you're enjoying what you're doing. If a man senses you're not enjoying yourself, he's probably not going to like it much, either (unless there's something very wrong with him, in which case you wouldn't be with him, would you).

The head of the male penis is extremely sensitive, when erect, so focusing too much on this at first is always going to be a mistake. You want to pay it adequate attention, but men like a bit of build up, so using your hands on the shaft, as well as your tongue and lips. Circling with the corona (penis-head) with the tongue is a perennial favorite.

Once the action has become a little hotter, you can use your lips on the corona, keeping your teeth covered and applying pressure with your lips as you take it in and out of your mouth. This movement mimics the sensation of the penis entering the vagina and men absolutely love it (including me and wife has it nailed). Don't be afraid to slobber. We not only don't care, we love it! Using this movement in conjunction with one hand sliding up and down the shaft creates a world of sensation, but remember to vary your moves when performing fellatio, as the penis can lose sensation if over-handled.

In essence, one good way to avoid triggering the gag reflex is to give up on the idea that a good blowjob means deep throating. While that can be fun; it's not necessary. You can show your man just as good a time without resorting to it, by employing some of the moves discussed here. If, however, you're determined to conquer that pesky gag reflex, that process starts in your mind.

Mind over gag reflex

The most important thing for women to remember, if they're serious about being able to deep-throat their partners, is to breathe through the nose. In deep fellatio, the penis actually enters the esophageal passage. If a woman is breathing through her mouth and not her nose, this will result in an inability to breathe. She may even vomit, which can be dangerous. It's not difficult to learn to breathe through the nose and women may find that practicing this form of breathing also serves to further relax them.

The simplest way for the penis to be deeply inserted in fellatio is for the giving party to have the head thrown back. This creates a direct passage between the mouth and esophagus, which is straight and not bent at the chin (as it is if the penis is approached in a kneeling position). Women will find that laying with their heads thrown back, with their partners entering from behind will be much easier, because the passage is straight and the muscles are more relaxed, as they're not engaged in this position.

Learning to relax the throat muscles is another important technique that can help with gag reflex. This can be achieved through slow entry, as well as intentionally breathing through the nose, while this is going on. In the position described above, the relaxation of these muscles will come much easier.

At this point, it's important for me to say that men who have partners with gag reflex problems need to be sensitive to that challenge if they want their partners to be able to engage in deep fellatio. Thrusting like a jackrabbit is going to ensure you never get what you want, so don't do it. Let your woman guide the action. Make sure she feels comfortable and trusts you with this activity, too. Don't blow it (pardon the pun) by losing control of yourself. She may never try again and it will be your fault.

Remember that slow and steady wins the race and that both partners have to be sensitive about overcoming the gag reflex problem. That means talking about it before you even think about attempting getting around it. If a woman's problem with fellatio has other origins (perhaps a bad or coercive experience), then it's of the utmost importance that she discusses this with her partner and trusts him enough to do so. Talk is the couple's road to sexual freedom and this is certainly true when it comes to enjoying oral sex together.

Time for the boys to go downtown

My lover loves me. Part of the reason is that I'm a cunnilingus (oral sex performed on a woman) specialist. That's because I love it. I have always loved it. I have always insisted on providing the service (even pre-love of my life) to my lovers and I have always actively sought to become more adept at its practice.

If you're a man who loves women, then you'd better learn to love going downtown. If you have a problem with it, I submit that you may have other issues that need to be discussed with your partner. Get to the bottom of it. Deal with it and then, be a man about it. If you want her to go down on you, you'd better be ready to go down on her and not in a half-hearted way, either.

That delicious flower between your woman's legs is a

complex thing of great beauty and sensitivity. The clitoris (that hyperactive little button that crowns the vaginal opening and extends down its sides, cushioned inside the labia, or lips) has more nerve endings in it than any other part of the human body – male or female. It is much more sensitive than the corona and, when aroused, can be the source of great pleasure for your partner.

The clitoris is to be approached with the utmost care. Like the corona, it can be shocked by too much attention, or attention that is too focused or brusque. The rule of thumb is don't be all thumbs. The clitoris, when you think about it, is a microcosm of the wondrous mystery that is "woman" in all her glory. Uniquely sensitive and luscious, this is the heart of your woman's sexuality.

Part of your sex play should be the downtown trolley. If you're not comfortable with that, then get comfortable with it. Now. Oral sex, prior to intercourse, is the most reliable way of getting your woman off. Going downtown before intercourse can also ensure that she has an orgasm during intercourse, also. If you play your cards right, you too can be the greatest lover ever known. Going downtown the right way is your ticket to that exalted status.

Becoming "Mr. Downtown"

As I've said, the clitoris is the most sensitive part of the human body (male or female); so approaching it with care is *de rigeur*. On top of that, it's important to remember that it's not the only part of a woman's genitalia. There's a lot going on down there, so learning to navigate all those sexy bits and pieces is going to make you a much better lover. The labia, because they contain the rest of the clitoris (what we call the "clit" is only the part that's visible), are also highly subject to stimulation with the lips and tongue. The vaginal opening is also part of her body that will respond extravagantly to your ministrations.

The clit itself must be dealt with delicately. As a matter of fact, over doing contact is exactly the wrong approach to take. A gentle flicking of the tongue, or a figure eight motion is your best bet. Intermittent blowing will also drive her absolutely wild. You may know all this, but perhaps you're rushing through it, or applying too much pressure. If that's the case, back off a bit and apply only the most delicate touch to this ultra sensitive part of her body.

Mastering cunnilingus is also a great way to take a break from intercourse, when you feel you're getting to the point at which you're finding it difficult to hold back. Concentrating on her orgasm for awhile is a great way of delaying your own and yet another way of showing her you're alive to the fact that mutual orgasm is something that matters to you, as her partner.

If you're a guy who doesn't even want to try cunnilingus, maybe that's because you have some anxiety about your performance. Nobody is born knowing everything. Everything in life, even walking and talking, has a learning curve attached to them. Lucky guys like me seem to have been born with silver tongues. That's great for me. It doesn't mean, however, that you're hopeless. You are in fact, a much better candidate for becoming Mr. Downtown than your fellows who aren't reading this book and who aren't interested in learning any new moves, because they think they've got them all. You are way ahead of the game just because you're here.

Your first and most important lesson is to learn that you can do it and you can do it to your partner's satisfaction. There's more than one way to skin a cat, but it's important that you stick to a few important ground rules, when it comes to upping your downtown game:

- Don't go in with all guns blazing. Gentle touch is what you're doing. Very little contact is always best.

- Don't lick. It's not an ice cream cone. The tip of your tongue, applied lightly is what you're doing.

- Don't put your teeth anywhere near the clitoris. That means not sucking it with the teeth in contact. I've heard stories about this and couldn't believe them, to be honest. So if you think this is a no brainer, then know that there are those out there who apparently have no brains and that's why this is being included.

- Don't pull at the labia with your hands to make the clit more accessible. This is wrong. Don't do it. Gently clear away any public hair in the region. The labia will take care of themselves. If you're worried about getting your chin wet, there's a problem.

Finally, if you genuinely have a problem with performing cunnilingus on your woman, then you have a problem showing her that you love her and care about her orgasm. If that's the case and you aren't dealing with it and don't care enough to deal with it, then you're not being the kind of man your woman deserves. Someone else will step up, if you won't. You heard it here first. (But if you've heard it before, then maybe it's time you listened).

Chapter 13: Manual Sex

"You need hands to hold someone you care for
You need hands to show that you're sincere"
(Lyrics: Max Bygraves)

Two hands. Five digits on each. That means ten whole fingers! Think of the possibilities our little mittens represent, so ripe with erotic potential. And yet, we don't do nearly enough with this expressive part of our bodies when it comes to getting it on.

Maybe we've all just forgotten how much fun they can be. Remember when they were all we had (especially you men)? I sure do. It was pretty cool to graduate from the lonely ignominy of solitary lovin' to actually having another person in the room with me for my erotic adventures. Of course, that evolutionary leap was also all about the hands, as they rushed and roamed over the bodies of my pubescent partners, longing to be followed by my other "digit".

We all remember with no little affection those early days of our sex lives, before that magic moment when we got naked with someone for the very first time. Our hands did most of the talking for us. Shy kisses having graduated to heavy petting, you could find us in the back row of the darkened movie theaters of America, hands busily exploring what we didn't yet have license to see in its totality. And then, of course, there were was the furtive fingering in the back seat of the car, not long after, and the Old Fashioned behind the football bleachers or bike sheds, after school.

Our hands, once we reach sexual maturity, seem not to have quite as much fun as they do in our callow youth. Not so much dangling at our sides, unused, they are sidelined somewhat, as the rest of our bodies are suddenly released from their juvenile prohibitions. We forget about our old buddies, as we lurch into the world of sexual maturity, penises ever at attention, vaginas ever emitting the "come hither" musk of availability, in the age of the birth control pill.

But there's really no need to neglect our tactile little friends. They can be part of the fun we're having with our lovers, too and they can make that fun even more varied and layered. Sure, we all use them during the course of our sex play to caress and touch, but do we really use them the way we did when had little other sexual recourse?

I think not. And I think, further, that it's incumbent upon us to do a little sexual regression therapy at this point and remember the days of our lives during which our hands were our primary form of sexual expression.

Your milkshake. Does it bring all the boys to the yard?

A lot of women wonder what the point of a hand job is. Why do some men like them so much? Well, a lot of that has to do with nostalgia. While it's true that our youthful sexual experiences are redolent of desire and erotic promise and thus, hold a special cachet for all of us, this may be doubly true for men. Many of us hold hand jobs in high regard for this very reason. They take us back to more innocent times; times when you weren't supposed to be doing "that". Any of that. And so, for men, the classic "Old Fashioned" is a rare treat, bearing with it our nostalgia for a youth, if not misspent, at least spent in the pursuit of the mysteries of our budding sexuality.

So, women readers, while you may never understand why it is men are so attached to this vestige of yester year, you should probably revive your chops, just for the sake of the sheer joy your partner will derive from you springing this relic on him every now and again.

The anatomy of an Old-Fashioned

The first thing you're going to need to make this operation go smoothly is, of course, a good lube (we'll talk about some of my favorites varieties later on). In the absence of lube (which I hope is not a regular occurrence in your household), a natural oil like coconut will do the trick. Unscented hand lotion is also a reasonable option. This last one may actually be particularly erotic for your male partner, particularly if you can (in a roundabout way) find out which one he was in the habit of having on his bedside table as a teen. Can you imagine his surprise, when you whip out a bottle right before treating him to an Old Fashioned? Such a plot twist might actually serve your efforts rather well, if I know men as well as I think I do. All the same, for the smoothest possible gliding action, a sexual lubricant is your best bet.

Once you've made it clear where you're going, you may want to up the ante by pretending to be his high school sweetheart. Giggle seductively as you whisper in his ear, asking him what time his parents are getting home. Watch the effect that has on him! Now wrap your well-lubricated hand lovingly around that effect and get to work with a few languid strokes.

Your grip should be firm. Our penises are pretty sturdy and squeezing them is something we truly enjoy. Don't be afraid to grip the shaft tightly, maybe checking in occasionally to make sure you haven't gone too far. Asking him can be fun, too. "Am I doing this right?" is a question we love to hear you ask. The answer may be pornographic, but that's all part of the fun, right?

Try placing both your hands on the shaft of your partner's penis. One hand can be placed on top of the other, with the top hand encircling the penis, just under the corona. Using your forefinger and thumb, form a ring and use this to slide and up and down, from just under the rim of the head, as the other slides up and down the shaft. You can also lace the fingers of your two hands together, wrapping both hands around your partner's penis.

A great way to vary the action is to remember the scrotum. Poor little scrotum is often ignored in the course of the Old Fashioned and this is a dreadful pity, as the male scrotum is alive with sensation. Unlike the shaft of the penis, the scrotum is quite sensitive and demands a light touch. Gentle cupping and tugging are in order. Using lube, you can also gently stroke the scrotum. As we've detailed earlier, the perineum is right behind the scrotal sack. This area is also ripe for stimulation, so gently massaging this as part of the fun is in order.

If your man is amenable (and I know not all men are – some of us are a little weird about our back doors), stimulation of the anus is also something worth exploring. Some of us really like this and (guess what) we're not all gay. There are loads of nerve endings in there, so if he's down (and you've discussed it beforehand – see what I did there), lube up and don't be shy.

Some of my readers might even want to ask their partners to show them how they do it themselves. No one has a better handle (yes, I said it) on what works than the handler-in-chief and that is your partner. Enjoy a show! What could be more instructional?

Five fingers to ecstasy

Unlike men, most women will have very little nostalgia for the pubescent manual efforts of early lovers. For many women, the build up to the actual groping was probably the most erotic part of the whole affair, with their youthful Romeos eventually modelling the manual dexterity of addled primates. Even with opposable thumbs, there is nothing quite as inelegant as a teenaged boy.

Who knows, though? Perhaps your female partner experimented early in life with those of her sex? It wouldn't be the first time in history! While the same may well be true for a lot of male readers, knowing the incredibly sensitive nature of male sexuality (being a male myself), I have spared you. Say thank you.

Nonetheless, manual sex for women requires an entirely different approach. Men need to be aware that approaching women's genitalia with our big, hairy mitts is not something to be taken lightly. In fact, there is some preparation involved, which is crucial.

A lot of men work with their hands. If that describes you, reader, please take a look at your hands, right now. What do you see? Are they as clean as they should be? Are the nails cut and filed? Are they hangnail free? Are they rough? According to your responses, it's incumbent on you to take appropriate, remedial action before you even think about getting those hams near your partner's lady parts.

I'm not asking you to sit down for a manicure. I'm asking you take a little time to take care of your hands, if you plan on going on this manual sexual adventure with your partner. She doesn't want you coming at her with hands that look like they've been rooting in the underbrush for days on end. Your hands need to be presentable and free of any rough edges that might possibly present a problem.

As with the Old Fashioned, "finger-banging", as we referred to it back in the day, was one of the few activities available to us young folk, without running afoul of the sexual prohibition which hung over many of us in our youth. While we all eventually broke the unwritten rules in one way or another (or all of 'em), we all remember rounding this particular base for the first time.

My women readers are probably staring off into space right now, remember that kid who first fumbled his way into her knickers back in middle school. I'm willing to bet that most of you are not smiling, either. As I've mentioned, teenaged boys aren't known for their manual dexterity, by and large. Some of you may have been fortunate enough, though, to have met your local high school's budding lothario – expert in the manual arts. Lucky you. You are the exceptions.

But we're all grown up, now. So for women, manual sexual exploration can be a revelation of this facet of sex and how much fun it can be in the company of a grown man; a man who doesn't employ his digits as though searching for an item he's lost up there, somewhere. Grown men know that women don't care to be handled like bowling balls. So let this be the first of my recommendations – women are not bowling balls. Govern yourselves accordingly.

I bet I can guess which color underwear you have on!

Men will happily entertain the idea of an Old Fashioned as a stand-alone activity. They will greet the prospect with great glee and anticipation. Women, however, when confronted with the same prospect, may view it somewhat differently. As I arrived at this section of the book, I decided to ask my partner why that was.

She thought about it for a moment and then told me that it was exceedingly rare to find even a grown man who had any clue as to how to approach the female genitalia with his hands. I'm happy to say that I was noted as an exception. I happen to know, however, that I am an exception only due to years of applied practice and practice and the gentle and patient guidance of my partner. Based on her feedback, I'm offering these tips for males looking to manually stimulate their partners, but from a completely different perspective – that of foreplay, shot through with role play.

If there's one thing we all know, it's that women enjoy extended foreplay. They want to feel good and revved up for the "main" event. Where women are concerned, it's all the main event and that's where they have most men beat. Women embrace sex in its fullness for what it is – sex. They don't prescribe to the Bill Clinton school of sex (which is intercourse, which is basically the global male attitude). Women see sex as a panorama of diverse activities, all constituting sex. The same is true for the manual stimulation of their genitals.

Women are looking for a male touch that mimics their own, in this regard. Just as we would like our female partners to grip our penises more confidently and without reservation (just as we would), they want us to touch their clitorises, labia and vaginas somewhat more tentatively and with some reserve and delicacy (just as they would).

That means giving yourself a pretext to go there. One way to do this is to harken back to those distant days of backseat groping, only on a decidedly more adult level. You may want to let your hand wander to her thigh, as you're sitting on the couch together, or perhaps at the movies. Whisper in her ear something saucy, like "I bet I know what color underwear you have on."

This will evoke a giggle. As your hand wanders up her thigh, she will probably demurely stop you, still giggling. But if you amp up your talk, you will amp up the intensity. Depending on your setting, this can go any way you finesse it to and it can go on for a very long time. If you're alone, you can even ask her to show you her underwear. Maybe ask your partner to sit on your lap, as you examine them and confirm your guess as to their color.

From here, gentle manual explorations (the way the you used to as a teen, only much less desperate) can be pursued, with the underwear still in place. Whether you've come to the car in the underground parking lot, following the movie, or are sitting on the couch, push the action along until you've reached the point at which you can ask to put your hand inside her underwear, perhaps pushing the crotch to one side, or pulling them down a little to accommodate skin-to-skin touching.

You can even ask your partner not to wear underwear, if you're going somewhere and tell her why, as you're on way there. Tell her what you have planned for later that evening, in the hall, in the upstairs washroom at the party, or in the darkened movie theater – in the back row. You're just horny school kids again, exploring each other for the first time, with your busy little hands.

Some women will be good and ready for digital penetration if you pursue the project in this way. Make it an adventure. Make it sexy. Appeal to her imagination and sense of fun. What was her nickname in high school? Find out and make sure you call her that, while you're playing your little game. What was her first boyfriend's name? Ditto. Going all the way can be over-rated when you and your partner are able to enter into a private world of sex play that's just as exciting and can be indulged in anywhere, any time. Just imagine the little smirks you'll walk around with after your session of finger banging! Naughty, naughty!

Key points to remember – your hands need to be beyond presentable and hygienically prepared. Your touch needs to be gentle and she has to be well lubricated. If you're saying the right things and you've set up the action well, that won't be a problem. And just as with the Old Fashioned, asking your partner for a private show will not only help you understand what her moves are with respect to her own genitalia, but can be highly erotic for both of you.

Chapter 14: Personal Lubricants

Here's where you're going to spend a few bucks, my friends and yes, it's worth every penny. The return on investment for these goodies is about as high a yield you'll get for any investment you'll ever make. And remember what you're investing in – your relationship and re-discovering the passion you've had with your partner in the past. Your love is worth it and your sex life, with the help of a little slippery fun, will be that much more joyous and thrilling.

We've talked about the usefulness of additional lubrication. I know a lot of people will think it's not necessary, or that there are household items which can just as easily be used, but that's not necessarily the case. Don't forget that you have to wash those sheets, towels, the rug, the curtains, the silk boxers and anything else lube comes into contact with. But part of the fun of lubrication is the fact that you have to go out, select and buy it and that such selection and purchase amounts to a pre-meditation of your mutual pleasure. What could possibly be sexier than going shopping together to find just the right lube? A shopping expedition *a deux*, followed by a private product demonstration. What fun! Let's talk about some of the various types of lube and what they're best suited to.

Slippin' and a slidin' – the lubrication basics

There are so many activities that lube can make better. Any kind of sex act is rendered much more sexual by the simple act of doing it with lube. So what if you don't need it? More is more! This is sex, people and you want it to be as sensual and lascivious, as slippery and as slidey as you can possibly make it. Being conservative about sex is a bit of a contradiction in terms, if you ask me. Go for the gusto!

Like a machine, when various body parts rub together, friction may occur which inhibits the optimum operation of the machinery involved. To keep everything ticking along seamlessly and without operational breakdown, machines often need to be properly oiled. Human beings have similar needs.

While the human body creates its own versions of sexual lubrication (in the uncircumcised penis and in the vagina, when aroused), sometimes, we want a little more of it. Or perhaps, we'd like some lubrication where it's not naturally produced. There are different kinds of lube and this is the first and most aspect of personal lubricants we're going to discuss, sub-genres not excepted.

Water-based

Most people prefer lubricants that are water-based for good reason – they're easier to clean up after. Getting water-based lube on your sheets isn't a catastrophe. Just throw that mess in the wash and be done with it! Same for your body – this type of lubricant washes off easily.

Water-based lubricants are also kind to the skin, as the water used in them is purified. Some lubes, also, can represent the danger of a condom breaking by degrading the latex these are made of. Most of you reading this are in long-term relationships, so I'm assuming you're not using these, but one never knows. It's good information to have at your disposal.

Silicon-based

This type of lube is beloved by many for its texture, which has a sensual, silken quality. Also, extremely good for those with sensitive skin are that silicon-based products that are hypoallergenic. Lubricants made with silicon are also known for their long duration. That means you'll have "re-load" less frequently than you might with a water-based lube.

All that said, the one thing about this type of lube is that it's not advisable for use with sex toys that are made of silicon, as this can cause the material to deteriorate. But take heart, because silicon-based lubricants are ideal for use when you and your love are going aquatic. In the shower, tub, lake, river or hotel swimming pool, silicon-based lubricants are ideal for water sports.

Hybrids

Just like the cars! Hybrids are a little bit water and little bit silicon, which means they can use them in water, too. While maintaining the naturalism of water-based products, they maintain the quality of longer duration that silicon-based products are known for. As with the 100% silicon type of lube, though, these are not good for use with any toys you might have, if you want to keep them in the best possible shape.

Oil-based

Some people really enjoy the sensation of an oil-based lube. Also good for sensitive skin, the heavier quality of an oil-based product can be uniquely sensual. That said, these lubes are not great for use with condoms. Latex doesn't much like oil. As said above, my long-term relationship readers may or may not care about this detail, but it's important safety information I feel it's responsible to include here.

Another important point about oil-based products is that they make a mess. So, if you're a fan, you may want to lay a couple of towels down on the bed before you get rolling.

If you've never used a sexual lubricant before, experiment with quantities. Start with a little and add more, if the two of you feel you need it. A little dab will do you isn't just for hair gel, or pomade. This maxim applies equally to lube. It's not exactly cheap, so start small and work your way up from there.

Personally, I'm a huge fan of hybrid lubes for their versatility. My partner and I are water sport enthusiasts, especially when we visit our favorite vacation rental (in an unnamed land), which features a private dipping pool. There's nothing like cooling off after a hot day at the beach with a hot evening in the dipping pool, a refreshing beverage and a side of long duration lubricant. For our toys, though (which we'll talk about shortly), we always use the time-honored water-based lubricant, as we like our toys and want them to enjoy long, happy lives.

My love and I are also fans of any product that warms upon application, as these can add an entirely new dimension to sex play. These are offered over a wide variety of product lines and price points. I suggest you do your research and find the one that's most appealing. Another "best practice" for happy couples everywhere, is carrying portable lubes. These are sachets that can be carried in your wallet or purse and put to work wherever you may be when the mood strikes you. Well worth the small investment required, these babies come in mighty handy in a pinch.

Lube is a chemical substance subject to deterioration in extreme temperature conditions, so like perfume, make sure to store it in a place which is subject to few fluctuations in temperature. You may find that you've soon accumulated a "lube cellar", so give your personal lubricant the respect it deserves and it'll be ready for playtime, when you and your love need it.

Where to buy it

You can buy personal lubricants pretty well anywhere, including on the internet. A trip to your local megastore or drugstore could send you home with what you need, too. A trip to Costco could send you home with enough of it for the entire neighborhood! But where's the fun and adventure in such mundane solutions?

I have a better idea!

You and your love will go on a shopping expedition. Every town on the map, these days, features at least one sex shop within shooting distance. If yours is a particularly pokey little town, with only one horse and no such retail outlets, then perhaps a weekend getaway to the nearest outpost of Western Civilization is in order? Re-discovering the passion you once shared as a couple is all about adventure and this could be one more. Plan your excursion, whether it's in your town, or to a nearby city. Make a shopping list together. Plan your adventure as you would any other excursion.

Once you've decided on the type of lube you'd like to experiment with, write it at the top of the list. I'm about to add to that list, with my personal recommendations of some of the best sex toys and "peripherals". These recommendations are all based on personal preference and incorporate the input of my love, because we've been on more than one such shopping expedition. We love doing this, from time to time, whether in search of something new, to find a specific product, or just to replenish our "lube cellar".

Let's jump into the world of sex toys with both feet. I was once a newbie in the land of the battery-operated sex prop, so if you're shy, I understand. It was, in fact, my adventurous partner who first dragged me into this exciting world and so, I'm returning the favor and inviting you along. Load in those batteries, kids! You're going to need them.

Chapter 15: A Madcap Adventure (In Ye Olde Sex Shoppe)

Once my love and I had established that the thrill had gone and had talked, at length, as to how we might invite it back, the lid was off the cookie jar. The lid never went back on, because we never found it again. It just disappeared, never to be seen again. The cookie jar was wide open and replenished frequently and with relish.

Not long after we started on our life long adventure as a couple dedicated to guardianship of the eternal flame burning between us, my partner broached the question. We were already well into the land of lubricants, but she was curious about other helpful items and wanted to explore them with me.

I was a little taken aback. Was I, her manly man, not enough for her? Was I somehow deficient? ("Is she going to come at me with a strap-on", was the question really on my mind).

She rolled her eyes and smiled wickedly. "Let's go on an adventure." To this day, that is her favorite word and something I dearly love her for, but it took me awhile to catch her enthusiasm and to feel comfortable with it. I guess I really started to relax once the strap-on was taken off the table (once and for all). Heaving a sigh of masculine relief, I started to like the idea and joined in seeking out the gizmos and wizmos that were going to make our sex life even more fun than it already was.

And so we hit the interwebs, poking around in what we thought were going to be some rather dark corners. And sure, there were dark corners. We saw things we can't unsee. We also saw that the world of sex toys has changed since the days of the plain, brown wrapper. In fact, the global sex toy market is now a $15 billion going concern, projected to grow into the triple digits by 2020.

That's a lot of dildos!

What that figure means is that the use of these peripherals is now as mainstream as, well, lube. Even when we were doing our research (about 8 years ago), we found that there were legitimate businesses which were not at all engaged in the promotion of pornography, peep shows, or anything more shady as better sex for people like my partner and I.

And so, we began to make a list. Each of the items we selected we agreed on as being of interest to both and not just one of us. We arrived at a budget for our shopping expedition, with a target date. We set up something like a critical path (she's fond of those). We were relentlessly organized about the whole thing and it became a private joke between us.

"ST minus 5", she would say. (Translation: sex toy expedition in five days).

"Copy." I would smirk back.

We're lucky to live in a fairly cosmopolitan American city, in which there are numerous purveyors of sex toys for middle class dabblers in the erotic arts, like ourselves. None of these is in "dodgy" parts of town. None of them has anything but a sterling reputation and all of them advertise in the hippest local newspapers, carried under the arm of every hipster in town, on the way to Saturday brunch.

And, after some deliberation, taking into account logistical concerns like closest transit hub and nearest pub for sex toy expedition post-mortem (with intermittent cackling), we chose our destination.

Owned by a lesbian couple and located in the trendy warehouse district, we liked everything about it, from the brick façade, to the granola-flavored, birkenstockian vibe of the neighborhood. It had horny old Hippie written all over it and that made us feel, somehow, like heirs of the ancients who once capered in Lincoln Park, flowers in their hair and pepper spray in their eyes.

And so, donning comfortable footwear and sleek urban getups, we ventured forth on our sex toy adventure, now freed from the bonds of bourgeois, uptight sexual convention. (Although the threat of the strap-on loomed in my lurid, male imagination).

From the ALRT to the bus to the sidewalk, to a stop at the obligatory coffee hub, we were there within the hour, standing outside, sipping our weekend lattes and peering through the discreetly dressed windows. We hovered. We giggled. We pointed.

Looking up, my eyes met those of what had to be one of the proprietors. Her bi-focals perched near the end of her nose, she resembled one of my long dead aunts – except for the hair, which was phosphorescent green and chaotically arranged on her head in an approximation of an updo. She smiled, waving me in. I reached out to touch my partner on the shoulder, never breaking eye contact with the green-haired woman waving at me from inside. My lover's fascination with the mysterious, egg-shaped object in the open, velvet box in the window broken, she followed my gaze. I could see her waving from the corner of my eye. Lattes in hand, we went inside.

She of the green hair was, indeed, one of the enthusiastic proprietors. A wealth of information, Shalene was all about sharing her intimate knowledge of her products with us, the uninitiated. She showed us items we'd only seen in the wilds of the interwebs and were unwilling to believe actually existed in the real world. But then, we saw them with our own eyes.

Bells, whistles and rotating bits abounded and as we became more comfortable with our surroundings (courtesy of the warm and inviting Mother of All Sex Toys, Shalene), we began to check off items on our carefully curated list. Shalene was only too happy to help us narrow down our selections and even suggest some fitting substitutions for some of what we'd written on our less-than-well-advised (yet ever so well intentioned) wish list.

And so, without further ado, I'm going to share with you some of our personal little friends as examples of the kind of fun stuff you can find out there in the sex toy market!

The Zini Deux

Looking not unlike a space age gaming peripheral, this interesting little gadget pulls apart to reveal vibrators that can be applied to both your fun zones. "His" and "hers" was never more intentional. The "hers" half stimulates the clitoris and labia simultaneously, while the "his" half does the same for his scrotum and associated areas. We love this doggone widget so darned much; we gave one to my lover's best friend for her birthday. She's used to us, so it was OK. (We haven't heard of it being re-gifted to any of the others).

Supersex Remote Control Love Egg

Imagine date night. A quiet, romantic dinner *a deux*? Perhaps soft music in the background. Wine, candlelight, holding hands across the table as you look into each other's eyes. But when you have the remote control to the love egg, your lover never knows quite what's next! Date night will never be the same when this little baby comes along for the ride. My partner hates to go to dinner without it and nobody has any idea she's even wearing it. Discreet, public fun for couples with shared secrets, who enjoy leering knowingly at one another in public places (as we do).

Five Smooth Stones

Sensual massage never had it so good, which means the two of you never have, either. This set of smooth rocks are heated and then, with the addition of ample lashings of massage oil, rubbed all over each other's body. Use your imaginations to put these deliciously sexy massage rocks to good use, rubbing each other the right way.

Ring a Ding Ding

All my readers will be somewhat familiar with the use of the penis ring. This device is intended to cause the penis to become harder and stay erect longer. It also provides the user with a much more intense eventual orgasm, due to the fact it helps you hold it off. The Lelo Tor is a highly sophisticated version of the classic penis ring, with an intense vibrating function to heighten the pleasure for both of you. As with any device of this nature, it pays to ensure that the one you're buying is the right size for you. Ask for the advice of your sage local sex shop owner.

Russian Hands, Roman Fingers

My partner and I fell in love with this one when Shalene drew it to our attention. We'd heard of such things, but believed them to be urban legends (even checking Snopes, at one point). But it's real and believe me, you're glad it is.

The Jimmy Jane Hello Touch is a fascinating device that will make you feel like 21st Century lovers, with shades of

Artificial Intelligence thrown in for good measure. Play robots, perhaps? Why not! The Jimmy Jane makes everything more fun. With two finger pads that extend from a power source located in a neoprene wristband, your imaginations (and fingers) will run wild, as the pads vibrate on any body part you place them on. The vibrations from the pads are powerful and serve to bring a whole new dimension to your foreplay game.

Fixsation

This one is intended to make female orgasm much easier! What could be easier than a little vibrator that is worn as a pair of underwear? Don't worry, gentlemen, it doesn't get in the way, but the vibrating element delivers vibrations in a variety of escalating intensities. The "underwear" detach from the vibrator, making it practical and easy to clean. My partner loves the Fixsation, as it's a fun addition to our repertoire, especially when we have to be some place and don't have a lot of time for buildup. This is a very useful little device we both derive a lot of pleasure from. It even comes in a super sexy satin pouch. A perfect gift!

Geek Appeal

I admit it. We're a little geeky. We can rhyme off whole sections of dialogue from any movie in the *Star Wars* franchise you'd care to name. We have even considered costumes, but we're still working on that one. For now, we have acquired a *Star Wars* vibrator.

That's right. We own a *Star Wars* vibrator. Don't be jealous!

Shalene had the full range (as her neck of the woods is ground zero for urban geeks, who tend to be rather enthusiastic customers, she relates). We decided on the Lord Vader. As the name suggests, this one looks a lot like the character from the films, which means that the "head" is wearing a helmet just like the one old Darth wears. You can just imagine how much fun we have with this one.

"Who's your daddy, Luke?" (Sorry).

Chapter 16: Home Décor for the Fun Loving Couple

Any fun loving couple will know that household furnishings and fittings have multiple uses. Couches aren't just for watching TV and kitchen tables aren't just for eating at. But there are, in our times, home furnishings made especially with your mutual pleasure in mind. These are attractive and discreet pieces of furniture that your parents won't even notice, except to perhaps remark upon how very attractive they are and where ever you found such an unusual item.

But sex furniture, truth be told, is nothing new under the sun. In fact, it goes back quite a ways, thousands of years in some places. While it doesn't seem that Catherine Great, the famous Russian Queen and sex enthusiast, had furniture designed to have sex on, she certainly had some other interesting items sitting around. These were discovered following World War II, when soldiers discovered a secret room in Catherine's former palace. In this room was a veritable treasure trove of erotic furniture, including an entire wall of phalluses, made from various materials. Tables and chairs depicted ejaculating penises, fellatio and cunnilingus were also found, some rendered in rather shocking detail. But Catherine was not the only crowned head of Europe who enjoyed a robust sex life and all the trappings that came with it.

Edward VII became King when his brother abdicated to marry his lover, Wallis Simpson. His exploits were famous throughout Europe, with women throwing themselves at him where ever he went. But Edward enjoyed the company of women who demanded pay for their efforts and so, was a regular at a famous brothel in Paris. He was, in fact, such a regular visitor, that a special suite of rooms was set aside for his exclusive use, even featuring the English royal coat-of-arms. In this suite was what would become one of the most notorious pieces of furniture in the world, and most probably the early prototype for today's sex furniture. This was Edward's *siege d'amour* (love seat). The famously obese king would engage on this seat with two prostitutes at a time, as it was easier for him to manoeuver due to his material physical dimensions.

If you're got a space in your house for one of the wonderful décor items descended from King Edward's early model, then I strongly advise you make a point of purchasing one. Let's talk a walk through the showroom and have a look at some of the better quality and more amusing pieces of furniture on the market.

The Wedge/Ramp

This one is a very important little helper that can provide the sort of elevation that makes sex a lot more comfortably effortless. Pillows are fine, but they tend not to retain their shape. They need to be continually fluffed as you're going along with the festivities, which can be both a distraction and an annoyance.

This firm, purpose-built wedge won't lose its shape. It will sturdily support you both, no matter how long you're on the job, or how many times you change positions. Best of all, it wipes clean! Useful, ergonomic and hygienic, too. We love ours. There's something about having something intentionally manufactured for your sexual use that is rather erotic. It's made the use of pillows in our house obsolete. Taking the wedge/ramp out of its discreet hiding place is a sign we're about to have a very special evening. I would highly recommend you add this one to your collection of sexual artifacts.

The Adela

This is a full-blown piece of furniture. Its futuristic lines are reminiscent of Kubrick's *A Clockwork Orange*, so if your home has a modernist theme, mom won't even blink when she first sees it. She'll just think it reflects your modernist aesthetic and perhaps sit on it, remarking that it's neither comfortable, nor practical. (This is the part where you and your partner exchange conspiratorial glances).

Named after the women who fought in Mexico's War of Independence, the Adelitas, the manufacturer puts a feminist spin on this accoutrement. Conjuring images of fierce Mexican women slung with bullet belts, their heaving breasts billowing from their cotton blouses as they kick the Spaniards out of their country, the Adela is for the woman who submits to no man.

Curvy and tricked out with foot rests and handles for leverage (that don't give themselves away at all, amazingly), you can tell your friends you bought this piece in a Chicago Gallery and that it is the new "Eames" chair. They'll nod thoughtfully, as they sip their snooty Chardonnay. You can feel good about the fib, though. This is a limited edition item and will run you rather a lot of dough. We have placed ours in a position of honor, in the front room, right in front of the Pollack print. It blends right in.

Wet Connection

This is another high-end item and one that is not to be taken at all lightly. This frosted glass shower stall is equipped with a series of cut outs, placed at various heights and arranged on its walls. Through these, the naughty possibilities are endless. If you're truly dedicated to fun in the shower, this is for you. Steamy showers *a deux* were never quite as much fun, especially if you're the type of couple willing to go to some expense to enjoy them in style. We are saving up for one. (Installation not included).

The Tantra Chair

Probably the most famous piece of sex furniture in the world, the Tantra Chair is an elegant, curvy piece of furniture worthy of any couple's living room – even in a place of honor. There's no need to squirrel this item away. It's that beautifully designed.

Covered in an eco-friendly composite material, which is also anti-microbial and very easy to wipe clean, the Tantra Chair is not only beautiful, but also sturdy and designed to last a lifetime. Its design echoes the human form and is made with optimum angles for lovemaking in mind. Using the chair makes sex easy, effortless and unique. Any position you can dream up is one this chair is going to take to its ultimate, ecstatic limit. Ours serves as our chaise, in discreetly located in the bedroom, but it might just as well be out in plain sight with the Adela.

Sex furniture's been around for a while and it can make sex a lot more fun. But it can also make sex a little easier for those who have physical limitations. People who have mobility issues and other physical challenges are rarely addressed in terms of information about sex and sexuality, so the next chapter in this book is about breaking that stigma. I really wanted to include this demographic and that's because of a personal experience of temporary disability I had not so long ago.

Chapter 17: Sex for People with Mobility Challenges

It seems that a lot of people don't really care to talk much about sex and mobility issues. In a world in which taboos are getting knocked down faster than pins in a bowling alley, that seems a little backward to me. Maybe that's because I've lived an experience of temporary disability and through that, have come to a fuller understanding of how that can play out in people's sex lives.

When I was scheduled for hip surgery, it hit me like a sledgehammer. I was too young. I was going to be completely helpless for as long as three weeks, using a walker. Then I'd be on a cane, learning how to walk with my new, bionic reality, all over again. I didn't relish the thought, but at the very least, I had a loving partner at my side to make the whole ordeal easier. When it finally came to attempting sex again, I learned what it was like to lose something, even if that loss was only temporary. This gave me a new respect and admiration for people who deal with disability and how that can impact their sexuality, every day of their lives.

When you go into the operating room, the last thing on your mind is sex. For one, you don't know if you'll ever wake up again. But once you get past that bit and you're on the mend – you remember that, yes – sex is good! You would like to have it again and soon. But what's a guy with a fresh hip replacement to do? It's counselled that you need at least six weeks prior to attempting sex again. In the meantime, there's always the Old Fashioned to keep you warm, not to mention the oral option, but your partner needs attention too.

For those with mobility issues, sex can be a challenge, but where there's a will there's a way, so this chapter's just for those of you who've either lost mobility temporarily, haven't had it for a while, or suffer from other physical challenges that make living out your sexuality a little more difficult than it is for most people.

The Ultimate Guide to Sex and Disability

This book is the exactly what it is says it is – a primer for those who live with a wide range of disabilities and challenges, but who continue to be enthusiastic about living out their sexuality. It's a comprehensive guide to sex, also, for those who suffer from conditions that cause them to suffer chronic pain (fibromyalgia), or chronic fatigue.

The book counsels the use of sex furniture, some of which is detailed in the previous chapter, like the wedge. This item can make sex a lot less physically stressful for those suffering from mobility issues, chronic pain, or both. While this may sound a little crazy, slings and swings are also a tremendous help for those who have physical limitations, or chronic pain. The weightlessness experienced in using these devices makes sex a stress and pain free operation. The Ultimate Guide enthusiastically counsels trying this solution when sex has taken a back seat to pain and/or disability and you're eager to get it back in your life. The Guide even gives "how to" instructions on how to make your own sex sling. Now, there's a worthy project for you and a special friend!

Sex after Multiple Sclerosis

Almost all of us have a friend or family member who suffers from this disease. Maybe it's you. Maybe it's your partner. What we know, though, is that MS touches all our lives, with 2.5 million sufferers worldwide and almost half a million in the USA, alone. Every day, almost 200 new cases are diagnosed.

Mimi Mosher is an MS patient who helps other patients get a handle on their sexual identities, following diagnosis. She believes that a healthy sexuality for MS people involves four crucial components, which are:

- Maintaining **confidence** in sexual identity is key for people with MS. A diagnosis can leave MS people feeling inadequate and insecure. Partners can certainly help with this side effect of the illness, as well as the family doctor.

- As I've tried to stress throughout this book, sex is a journey and it should be a fun one. That means that **exploration** part of the fun. For people with MS, whose nervous systems have been compromised by the disease, mobility issues may demand that partners are sensitive to the changes that can occur. Looking at sex from the perspective of intimacy (before gratification) can open the door to more satisfying sex for both partners. Instead of MS ruining the sex lives of couples in which one partner has the disease, it can broaden their horizons.

- As with any challenge that represents a change in mobility status, couples facing the challenge are called upon to **get creative**. Using lubricants that produce additional sensation, or employing vibrators and other means of enhanced stimulation can address a loss of sensation. Sex furniture can help, too. The key is an open discussion between partners about how you're going to meet the challenge and make it an exciting adventure you share together.

- All good sex demands **trial and error**. No one is born knowing how to be "good in bed". The challenge may be multiplied when MS is the third party in the bedroom, but that doesn't mean your curiosity should be stymied. It should, in fact, be stimulated by this new reality. Trying new things and letting go of those practices which no longer work for you is all part of what it means to be a loving couple, dedicated to one another's pleasure.

Men suffering from MS may have difficulty maintaining an erection, but this is not the end of the world, by any means. Problems with muscle cramps can also occur which make staying in the mood difficult. For this problem, the market is flooded with pharmaceutical aids that can help men maintain their erections. Also available are vacuum pumps and rings (as described in the chapter on sex toys). These are also helpful for women partners with MS, who have lost some of their libido, but aren't willing to let their partners go without.

Pain and a loss of lubrication are also problems women with MS may suffer from. The same de-sensitizing lubricants used by men to delay ejaculation can be used by women to reduce discomfort when having intercourse. There are many such products available and they can all be used safely by women. Personal lubricants can help replace natural lubrication lost to MS and pave the way for pleasurable sex, without the discomfort generally associated with such loss.

Finally, spasticity is a common problem for people of both sexes, with MS. This can be exacerbated by orgasm. To help avoid the occurrence of muscle spasms, massage is indicated. The act of massage is one of total, physical intimacy between partners. This activity can also be a substitute for intercourse at those times when it becomes difficult for one or both partners. By relaxing the muscles through prolonged massage (perhaps using a vibrator), partners can strengthen their bond and engage in a type of eroticism that is less demanding than more traditional methods of engaging in sexual activity. Massage is proven to reduce the occurrence of muscle spasms, thus making orgasm the pleasure it's supposed to be and not the problem it can be for people with MS.

No boundaries

Even my personal experience of temporary disability was difficult for me to absorb, as a man. Men suffer from a unique complex of insecurities centered on our sexuality that can make us extremely sensitivity to any perceived diminishment in our virility. Negative self-talk can take over, getting in the way of your sexuality and finally, killing it, as your sexual confidence takes a nosedive.

As I've written this book primarily for use by partners in long-term relationships and marriages, I'm going to address the same constituency here. A loving partner is a key ingredient for people with disabilities of any kind having a satisfying sex life. But a satisfying sex life is the birth right of all people and not only for those who have no physical challenges. That means that even people who are not partnered should able to live out their sexuality as fully as possible.

Whether this is done by autoerotic means (self-stimulation), or the use of sexual surrogates (people you can hire to assist you, sexually, dedicated to service to disabled people), it's the right of every living person to live out their sexuality.

Couples who support and love one another can find a way around any challenge or obstacle. In all the great love stories, love conquers all and that includes physical challenges like the loss of mobility, MS, chronic fatigue and chronic pain. When one of you is suffering, there is a world of help out there that you only have to look for and call on. Your life as a physically loving couple doesn't end with disability. It may, in fact, only be getting started.

Chapter 18: Would You Ever?

Sex is an endless kaleidoscope of possibilities. Just when you thought it was all getting a little tired, along comes another wrinkle in your sexual world, to shake things up again.

A wrinkle, or a kink?

Ah, there's that word. Kink is not all whips and chains. Kink can involve fetishization of certain types of clothing, or body parts, or even household objects. (Stop looking at the blender like that). Kink can be role-play, or public sexual behavior. It can be lots and lots of different things. For as many people as there are in this world, there are different types of kink and you know what? With willing partners, it's okay.

Sometimes people are awfully shy about admitting to a kink or fetish. That's because we live in a judgmental world. Something I've learned in my life, though, is that those who judge you are the people who are most likely to have a closet full of secrets; things they kept hidden, out of shame. But their shame is not your problem. Only your shame is your problem and the fact is that kinkiness is the human condition. There's nothing to be ashamed of.

Role play

You're a superstar. You know you are. You and your partner are the same people every day, doing more or less the same things. Sometimes, when the moment's right, its kind of fun to put aside our day-to-day personas and be someone else for a little bit. At least, I think it is. My partner does too.

We were on vacation at an all-inclusive beach resort when we found out just how much fun role-play can be. We spent that vacation mostly recharging our batteries, poolside. Cradling cool drinks in our languidly lazy (and sun browned) mitts, we were as indolent as the day was long, refusing to budge, except to dunk ourselves in the pool momentarily, or flag the waiter down.

And it was that waiter that broke the camel's back. My partner, much to my chagrin, couldn't keep her eyes off him. I admit that he was a pleasant looking guy (OK, he was built like a brick outhouse and had dimples you could stick your finger in up to the first knuckle). Finally, after observing her eyes peeping out over the top of her sunglasses to bore holes into the guy's ass as he walked away one too many occasions, I got a little testy.

"I can see you, you know." I snorted, sarcastically. "You're not invisible!"

Naturally, my partner pretended not to know what I was talking about, directing her attention back to her pulp fiction, poolside reading. As for me, I sat there turning the meaning of my partner's ogling ways over in my mind. After doing so for the better part of the afternoon, I began to formulate a plan.

When it was time to return to our room to shower and get ready for dinner, I pretended to have an errand to run. I wandered around the grounds of the resort for about twenty minutes and when I felt enough time had elapsed, returned to the room. Knocking on the door, I called out, "Room service!"

When my partner arrived at the door, she found me there, frosty cocktail, replete with paper umbrella, on a tray I'd managed to convince one of the guys at the swim up bar to lend me for the occasion. She'd just gotten out of the shower and had come to the door wearing a towel.
"Oh, pardon me ma'am! I'm so sorry to disturb you." My eyes roved up and down the length of her towel-clad body, as I said this, lingering on her breasts.

My partner's eyebrows shot up, as she cottoned on.

"That's no problem. Do come in". She pulled the door open, still hanging on to the towel. Closing the door behind me, she gestured to the table in the sitting area. "You can put that over there". And so I did. But when I turned around, my partner had dropped the towel to the floor at her feet and it was *on*.

Without so much as saying a word, I had become my partner's dirty little fantasy, come to life in our hotel room. It was as easy as paying attention to what was going on right in front of me and transforming it into an experience we could share and enjoy together. This is where putting aside uselessly hurt feelings comes into play. Why should you be hurt or even mildly annoyed that your partner sees other people as attractive? This is just a human thing and an indication that your partner is, in fact, still living!

Don't get angry. Get creative. Take that attraction and make it a game you can both get off playing. That's how the smart folks do things.

Bondage

A little light bondage can be very erotic. It just depends where you're both at, as to whether this option is going to work for you. I'm not talking about heavy-duty dungeon play. Then again, that might be your thing (which is another book, entirely). I'm talking about light restraints around the wrists and possibly, the ankles. This can work for either partner. Have a little chat. Find out if this is something your partner may like. I've found that springing things on my partner can work either for or against me, so once again, knowing your partner well is your best sexual tutor. You know who your partner is better than anyone. Let that knowledge be your guide.

Your visit to the sex shop can encompass this aspect of sex play, too. There are even kits available, which include everything from feather ticklers, to satin wrist restraints and blindfolds, to kinky little whips made of soft, non-threatening material. Perhaps making a gift to your partner of one such kit can break the ice. If such presentation concludes with something else getting broken, there's your answer.

Spanking

Spanking is a becoming an increasingly popular activity for fun loving couples. As with everything else in this book, its two-way street and one which both of you can enjoy giving and receiving. You may want to incorporate it into your role play, with one of you playing the principal to the naughty school girl/boy. Lights! Cameras! Action! You may even need costumes.

Spanking, though, needn't even incorporate any elaborate scenarios, or equipment. The flat of someone's hand and a naked bottom are quite enough. When incorporated into your sex play, a little slap on the bum can be powerfully erotic and you may find that you both become rather fond of the activity. The trick, of course, is knowing when you've gone a little too far. It's important, when engaging in any activity involving restraints or BDSM (bondage, domination, sadism, masochism), that you're both invested with the ability to stop the action if it's going beyond what you're willing to indulge. That means employing a safe word.

A safe word is what you say when you don't like the direction the action is taking. It has to be a word that neither of you would normally say in the course of your love play. For example, "Pythagoras" is a rather good one. Also appropriate might be a word like "cumberbund" (it's not as though either of you is going to be wearing one – generally speaking). Having an agreed upon safe word in place can also be fun at parties, when you're both ready to leave for the evening, or if you find someone to be a terrific bore, but don't dare say as much to his or her face. You can always explain it away as a type of Tourette's, if it comes off as too "weird".

Conclusion

What a wonder sex can be for a loving couple. When both partners are actively engaged in keeping the flame alive, sex can be the glue that binds them together. When we let that flame die, for whatever reason, our lives together lose something. We become roommates who used to find each other attractive, once upon a time and perhaps forget how that happened.

It can happen to anyone. It doesn't mean there's something wrong with you, or your partner. Letting the fire go out happens to most people, over the course of their relationships, but I'm here to tell you that the condition is not permanent. With some genuine commitment and sustained remedial action, you can light it up again and it won't even take that much effort. It just takes commitment, dedication and the love that's already there, between you and your partner.

That never went anywhere. That love is still there. It's like gasoline, waiting for a match to be dropped on it. Re-learning how to physically express your love is something the two of you can not only talk about, but do. You can do it together. If only one of you is coming along for the ride, then maybe the writing is on the wall. I'm the type of guy, though, who genuinely believes that if the love is real, then the sex is not dead forever. It's just taking a nap and needs a wakeup call.

With your unique, combined creativity as a couple, every day is going to be an adventure. Your willingness to explore and to rediscover the people you fell in love with, will have you falling in love all over again. There was a time when you couldn't keep your hands off each other and that time can be *now*, if you're willing to do what it takes to make it happen.

My partner and I, like almost every living couple, has been there. We've let the flame go out. But because we know each other so well and because we love each other so deeply, we've been able to not only revive our sexual relationship, we've been able to make it better than it was, even in our earliest days together. As we've grown together we've become stronger and more fully rounded human beings. Experience has taught us many things, as it teaches us all. That's the part about getting older that's beautiful. Life teaches you as you move through it and all that learning can enrich your lives together, emotionally, sexually and spiritually.

Your relationship was born in passion. There's no reason to believe it's not still there. In fact, believing that serves as the cornerstone re-discovering that passion, together. If your love is real, it was built to last and something built to last is worth keeping in the best shape you possibly can.

While life can throw us curveballs, wear us out and squash us down, our response to those challenges is what really makes the whole affair worth living. Being who you are together and who you've always been as a couple, is a shared adventure and sexuality is an important part of that. Whether you're young, old, physically unencumbered, or disabled, your sexuality is an integral part of your humanity. Living that out in all the fullness and joy sex brings to our lives is your birthright and your gift to one another.

I hope you've enjoyed this open, high-spirited discussion about re-discovering sexual passion as a committed couple.

More than that, though, I hope you take what I've written here to heart and that you and your partner can put it to the right kind of use – re-igniting the passion in your relationship. By doing that, you can be a light to other couples out there who may be floundering. The quality of your life having changed because of your dedication to each other, you'll stand as an example to others that love is not disposable. It may change, over time. But it's something worth defending and something worth spending the time to reinforce, by giving ourselves fully to each other. We were born for each other. Let's remember that, and live out our love with our bodies, minds and spirits. Let's be the promise we made to one another in the very beginning.

May you re-discover your passion for each other and live as lovers, always.

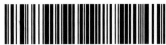

79349425R00072

Made in the USA
Lexington, KY
20 January 2018